Tao and Dharma

CHINESE MEDICINE AND AYURVEDA

Robert Svoboda and Arnie Lade

Foreword by
Michael Tierra, O.M.D.

LOTUS PRESS
PO Box 325
Twin Lakes, WI 53181 USA

DISCLAIMER

This book is a reference work, not intended to diagnose, prescribe or treat. The information contained herein is in no way to be considered as a substitute for consultation with a licensed health-care professional.

Cover design and drawing by Navaja B. Llope
Book design by Regan C. Mitchell

First Edition 1995
Printed in the United States of America.

ISBN 0-914955-21-7
Library of Congress Catalogue Card No. 95-80859

CONTENTS

ILLUSTRATIONS

FOREWORD

Traditional Chinese and Ayurvedic medicine constitute the two major legacies for health and healing from the ancient world. However, one distinction between the two is found in the fact that traditional Chinese medicine, as introduced to the West during the 70s and 80s represents a more physio-materialistic focus. This is because of the effort that was made to clear away its spiritualistic orientation so that it could better accommodate the tenets of Chinese Communist materialism. Ayurvedic medicine—which followed Indian yoga into the West and had no dominant ideology, such as Communism to modify it—maintains a closer integration with spiritualistic yogic philosophy.

As this book so aptly points out, while there are differences between the two great systems, the similarities are even greater. Is it, however, from a collective unconscious that two great healing arts, such as traditional Chinese medicine and Ayurveda arise, or is it from a primal source that extends beyond our present geographical and archaeological understanding?

Visiting a rainforest near Cairns, Australia, I was amazed to find species of plants identical to species that only grow in one other part of the planet, a particular area of the Amazon rainforest in South America. Just as we find identical or similar species of plants simultaneously growing today on distant and different continents throughout the world, is it not possible that universal knowledge and wisdom of humanity might have been preserved and passed on from one long-forgotten prehistoric source?

As with other ancient stories and myths of the world, the story of the Garden of Eden in the Book of Genesis offers an insight into the origin of consciousness. The eating of the forbidden fruit, rather than representing a fall from grace and innocence, signifies our innate thirst for greater knowledge which leads us into the consciousness of relativity.

Nothing escapes the gods of relativity; there can be no absolute good and bad, beauty and ugliness. Humankind must forever feel the inner compulsion or inspiration to find the positive in the negative and the oftentimes more difficult alternative of acknowledging the negative in the positive. This same relativity goes beyond the moral order, to find expression in the Taoist Yin-Yang philosophy and the three Doshas of Ayurveda, both of which formerly evolved and were used according to their respective cultural contexts to determine the most balanced and appropriate diet, herbs, exercise and lifestyle according to inherited constitution, life work and climate.

In these times of maximum fragmentation, it is truly a miracle that the perennial truths and the healing capacities of these great ancient philosophies can arise. As we usher in a new planetary order, we must proceed with both respect and caution as we find a new integration of the ancient wisdom and apply it to plants, climates and circumstances around the world.

To this purpose, this valuable work should serve as an important contribution.

Michael Tierra, O.M.D.

ACKNOWLEDGEMENT

The authors wish to thank James Williams, Michael Tierra and Fred Smith for their gracious reviews of this book during its development. Special thanks to Diane Lade for providing the fine illustrations of plants that appear in Appendix I.

INTRODUCTION

Chinese and Indian medicine embody the two oldest continuously practiced traditions of medicine on the planet. These traditions are oceans
of wisdom whose depth and breadth are almost incomprehensible to one
who stands on their shores. Into these oceans of healing art tributaries of
thought flow, and the two seas have at times mingled their waters together. Though the origins of these medical traditions have no fixed historical landmarks, they seem to have appeared at approximately the same
time, yet independently, grown out of an understanding expounded by
their sages and rishis. Centuries passed after Chinese and Indian medicine
were founded before they first mingled to exchange ideas with each other.
Why two great systems should appear simultaneously in two vastly different corners of the globe, each a unique expression yet possessing many
similar characteristics, is a great mystery. Perhaps their fundamental vision
and insights about life grew out of humanity's collective unconscious.

At the heart of both of these great healing traditions is a world
view which sees man and nature as inextricably linked. From this perspective each elucidates its own understanding of health, meaning of disease
and journey from illness to health, both employing analogies to the forces
and manifestations of nature to express their views. These insights were
carefully refined, systematized, clinically verified, orally transmitted and
later recorded in writing. Contained within the written traditions of both
systems are the experiences of countless physicians and patients which
serve today as an immense storehouse of knowledge.

The goal of this book is to convey to the reader an introductory
understanding of Indian (Ayurveda) and Chinese medicine, and to compare these understandings. Inherently Ayurveda and Chinese medicine
both explain, in their own terms, health and illness, and each offers direction for regaining health. Since they share much common ground each
can enhance certain themes and expand the vision of the other, and
hopefully through this work new ideas will emerge which can intellectu-
ally cross-fertilize students and practitioners of both systems. Perhaps ultimately these two energetic paradigms can be reconciled, not by a whole-
sale incorporation of one tradition into the other but, as has happened
over the centuries, by an exchange of ideas, techniques and principles.
Reconciliation will require that the proponents of both systems remain
open-minded, willing to reflect objectively on the strengths and weak-
nesses of their respective fields.

In both North America and Europe the past few years have seen a
dramatic rise of interest in Chinese medicine and Ayurveda. As these two
traditions establish niches for themselves as "alternative medical systems",
their practices will undoubtedly be modified by their new social, economic
and medical milieu. A thorough understanding of the Asian roots of these
two medical traditions is, we believe, essential to the success of their trans-

plantation here. Some hybridization may well be necessary to effect their successful propagation in the context of our modern days, since it is always difficult to transfer concepts from one culture to another, but we have tried assiduously in this essay to maintain intact the original meanings of the theories and practices so that their flavor will not suffer. The common tendency today in the West is to look at Ayurveda and Chinese medicine from a modern biomedical approach; we suggest that there is merit in comparing one with the other, since both are energetic in nature.

This book is divided into three parts. The first and second detail the basic theories and practice of Chinese medicine and Ayurveda, respectively, while the third consists of a comparative study of both systems, including an outline of what we know of their historical relationship with each other. Following the third part, a summary of our main conclusions is given. In addition two appendices are provided, the first outlines the history and use of twelve medicinal substances by both Chinese and Indian systems, whereas the second reviews the use of vital points in Asia.

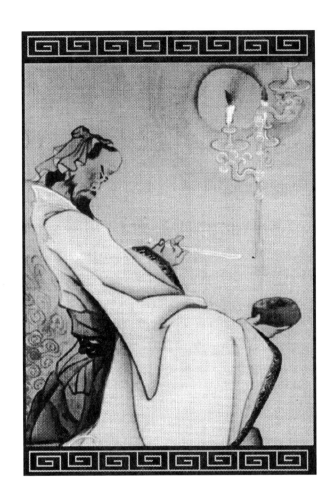

PART ONE
CHINESE MEDICINE

1
Origins and Development

A fundamental tenet of the Chinese system of medicine is that the human body-mind-spirit continuum is an integral whole, and that the individual is linked to a greater macrocosmic entirety through a progressive continuum from family, society, environment and, ultimately, the universe. From this perspective, the manifestation of disease is viewed as the outcome of an imbalance originating within oneself or in one's relationship to external reality. Conversely, health is a state of both internal and external harmony. Chinese medicine has since antiquity provided a clear description of these ideas, formulated principles for understanding their relationships, and developed unique therapies to correct imbalance.

The origins of Chinese medicine are clouded by the mists of time. Descriptions of some aspects of early medical practice in China are found in the *Historical Memoirs* (*Shi Ji*), which is the first book in a series of dynastic records written about 500 B.C., wherein the various forms of diagnostic procedures of pulse study, inspection of the tongue and methods for questioning are discussed, as well as the therapeutic modalities of acupuncture, moxibustion, massage, remedial exercise and the use of plant medicines.

The earliest medical text extant is the *Yellow Emperor's Inner Classic* (*Huang Di Nei Jing*) first appearing in the later part of the Warring States period (475–221 B.C.). The *Inner Classic*, which is still highly regarded and studied in all the colleges that teach traditional Chinese medicine, is a heterogeneous treatise which includes a summation of the different medical approaches and practices found at that time in China. It covers numerous topics, including the interpretation of disease, the physiology and pathology of the internal organs, and anatomy, including an understanding that the heart is the center of the blood's circulation. Many varied and seemingly opposed theories and practices, such as the Yin-Yang and Five Element doctrines, Taoism, Confucianism and shamanic healing, are all discussed. The ancient authors clearly felt no need to synthesize all the various traditions, or to propagate just one doctrine. Their effort was rather to attempt to reconcile opposing interpretations. This inclusion of sometimes antagonistic views and approaches is an early and enduring trait of Chinese medicine.

Subsequent works especially of the Han Dynasty (206 B.C.–220

A.D.) laid the groundwork for the system that has come down to us today. Three texts of this period stand out, the first being the *Classic of Difficult Issues (Nan Jing)* which elaborated and clarified the theories of the *Inner Classic*, especially on the correspondences and uses of Five Element doctrine and on the use of the wrist pulse for diagnosis. The second major work, *Discussion of Cold Induced Disorders (Shan Han Lung)*, summarized the prevention and treatment of infectious and febrile diseases, listing 370 prescriptions, while the third, China's first materia medica, *Shen Nong's Materia Medica (Shen Nong Ben Cao)*, recorded 365 different types of medicinal substances of plant, animal and mineral nature, noting their properties and effects. Today many such ancient texts are lost; nevertheless, there are more than 6,000 available texts recording the clinical experiences and evolving theoretical knowledge of Chinese medicine.

The Han Dynasty saw three great master-physicians: Zhang Ji who codified medical practices and wrote the above mentioned text, *Discussion of Cold Induced Disorders*; Chunyu Yi, a famous doctor and master of pulse diagnosis; and Hua Tuo, a remarkable surgeon, acupuncturist and inventor of a unique gymnastic exercise.

The appearance of these great classics occurred during the formative period of Chinese medicine. In this period Chinese medicine was taught and practiced systematically and was held in high esteem, gaining official sanction under various emperors. As far back as 165 B.C., the Chinese state regulated the licensing and education of physicians. Fifty years later the first imperial university was established, teaching such sciences as astronomy, hydrology and medicine. By the 7th century A.D., most larger provincial cities had government-run colleges of medicine. The golden age of Chinese medicine occurred between the 4th and 10th centuries, when public apothecaries and hospitals were founded, an official pharmacopeia was composed, foreign ideas studied, new methods developed, and new treatises written. It was during this colorful age that Chinese medicine defined itself into the form in which, with only slight modification, we see it today.

2
The Tao and Yin-Yang Philosophy

A n ancient Chinese master once said: "Writings do not express words clearly, words do not express thoughts clearly"; to which his dismayed disciple replied: "Then one cannot comprehend the thoughts of the sages." The Master answered: "Thus the sages created images in order to express thoughts clearly." This echoes the words of Lao Zi (circa 6th century B.C.), the grandfather of Taoism, in the first lines of the *Classic of the Tao and Its Virtue* (*Dao De Jing* or *Tao Te Ching*): "The Tao that can be told is not the eternal Tao; the name that can be told is not the eternal name."

The terms Tao, Yin and Yang are images fashioned by the ancient Chinese sages to describe their insights into reality. This love of imagery with a parallel affinity for vagueness and economy of words is reflected in all the classics, and in the Chinese pictographic writing system. In the Tao-ist view the word Tao is used to denote the all-embracing first principle, the eternal primordial source called also the Void, as well as the potential from which all things arise. In the passive state the Tao is empty and non-reactive, while in its active state the Tao is seen as universal progenitor which creates reality and keeps it together, functioning, vitalized and constantly changing, though the Tao itself remains unchanged. This is in accord with the ancient Chinese world view that all phenomena are interdependent. Additionally, the Tao infuses each thing with a unique Virtue or Nature (de), composed of both quality and force. Essentially an expression of the Tao, Virtue or Nature gives rise to all distinguishable patterns and forms.

The ancient sages placed great emphasis on trying to understand reality through the careful study of the patterns found in nature. Building upon the concept of Tao the ancients formulated a dualistic theory called Yin-Yang to describe and interpret these patterns manifest in creation. Lao Zi states: "The Tao begot one, one begot two, two begot three and three begot the ten thousand things; the ten thousand things carry Yin and embrace Yang and through their blending of forces they achieve harmony." This is an important metaphor used to describe primal images. The Tao referred to here is the passive Tao, the Void (wu), which gives rise to the one, the active aspect of Tao also referred to as the Supreme Ultimate (tai yi). From oneness a dualistic tendency arises in the form of Yin-Yang which in turn gives birth to three, the initial manifestation of energy as a third force: Qi. Three also symbolizes the fields of primal activity, referred to as Heaven, Earth and Man, and three is the minimum number of lines necessary to enclose space (as in a triangle). The phrase "ten thousand things" represents the diverse creation (see illustration 1).

The terms Yin and Yang, whose etymological roots refer to the dark and lighted sides of a mountain respectively, were gradually extended to refer to the principle of duality inherent in all manifestation. Yin and Yang's relationship to each other is one of vital, not static, duality. They are seen as two primal forces in a state of constant change, which the ancient divinatory text known as the *Classic of Changes* (*Yi Jing* or *I Ching*) calls the permanent condition of the universe. Underlying this perpetual flux and motion between the polar forces of Yin-Yang, which causing them to unite, transform, separate and regenerate, is the potential found in Tao. Again, in the *Classic of Changes* the concept of three, as in the triagram symbol, is an important image to understand space and reality.

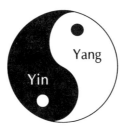

The images of Yin and Yang have at their base Nature, which in itself is an ever-changing phenomenon. The recognition of the orderly patterns in the celestial movements in the heavens above and in the cycles of the seasons on earth below provided early mankind with a way to measure and anticipate change. In both the ancient oracle inscriptions and the *Classic of Changes* the image of the receptive Earth below and the creative Heaven above form primary attributes ascribed to Yin and Yang respectively.

The *Inner Classic* uses the analogies of water and fire to describe the intrinsic attributes of their opposing natures, as summarized below:

WATER-YIN	FIRE-YANG
coldness	heat
moistness	dryness
dimness	brightness
downward & inward movement	upward & outward movement
stillness	activity
yielding	forceful
inhibition	excitation
slowness	rapidity
heaviness	lightness

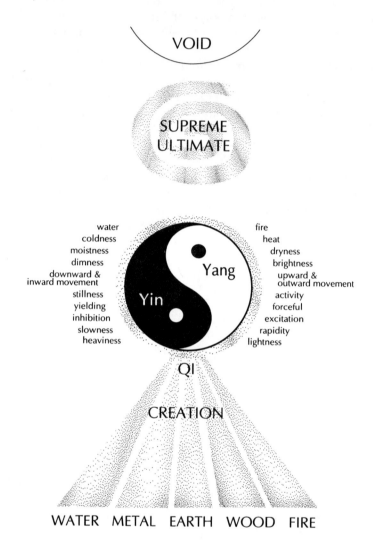

VOID

SUPREME
ULTIMATE

water
coldness
moistness
dimness
downward &
inward movement
stillness
yielding
inhibition
slowness
heaviness

Yang

Yin

fire
heat
dryness
brightness
upward &
outward movement
activity
forceful
excitation
rapidity
lightness

QI

CREATION

WATER   METAL   EARTH   WOOD   FIRE

1. Chinese Creation Philosophy

According to Chinese philosophy, from the Void (wu) arose the One or Supreme Ultimate (tai
yi) that generates the primal duality known as Yin and Yang. A third force, Qi, emerges from
the tension generated by the Yin-Yang polarity. Creation is seen as a result of the interplay
between Yin, Yang, and Qi. The Five Elements (wu xing) are derived from this cosmic play
and are used to understand and organize reality.

Practically speaking, four primary principles explain the dynamic relationship between Yin and Yang in traditional Chinese medicine:

1) All phenomena contain two innate opposing aspects.
2) Yin and Yang are co-dependent.
3) Yin and Yang nurture each other.
4) Between Yin-Yang there exists a transformative potential.

These basic principles governing the relationship between Yin and Yang are well illustrated by the traditional diagram of the Supreme Ultimate. The universe is symbolically composed of the primal forces of Yin and Yang, represented as black and white respectively, forming a unified circular whole. Within each colored half there is a contrasting spot indicating there are no absolutes and that both forces only exist in relation to each other, just as night-time exists only in relationship to day-time. The moving interface between the two halves denotes their vital nature and nurturing tendency, which in extremes can cause transformations to occur. The symbol also indicates the tendency of Yin-Yang towards balance, for their overall appearance is one of equal strength.

3
The Five Elements

Zou Yin (350-270 B.C.) is generally accepted by historians to have first formally articulated an integrated theory based upon the Five Elements (wu xing). He was a brilliant philosopher who combined the Yin-Yang doctrine with the Five Elements and is credited with developing an original method of induction used to interpret and predict human and natural affairs in an orderly way. The Five Element doctrine as an important secondary system of correspondences first had an impact on Chinese medicine with its inclusion in the *Inner Classic* and then more substantially in the *Classic of Difficult Issues*. The term "Five Element" is used here out of convention following the usage of other English texts on Chinese medicine, as well as to facilitate cross reference in approaching similar concepts in Indian medicine, but actually the characters translate more accurately as the Five Phases or Movements, for the Chinese were more interested in process and patterns than in substance and structure.

The five substances wood, fire, earth, metal and water specifically symbolize the fundamental qualities and behavioral patterns intrinsic to the universe. The attributes of the Five Elements are summarized as follows: Wood is characterized by the process of germination and a spreading outward tendency; Fire is an emblem for heat and growth with an impulse for flaring upwards; Earth represents transformation and nourishment with a tendency towards containment; Metal is characterized by the maturing process and a concentrating influence; and Water represents coolness, decay, transmutation and storage with a downward flowing motion.

There are two other important patterning methods within the Five Element model known as the Generative and the Control cycles (xiang sheng & xiang ke). The Generative cycle describes the inherent order of activity found amongst the Elements i.e. germination (Wood), growth (Fire), nourishment (Earth), ripening (Metal), and decay with the guarding and storage of the seed-essence (Water) which allows for the cycle to begin again at the germination stage. The annually repeated procession of the seasons, as found in temperate climates such as that of China, are a natural example of this concept.

The Control cycle, similarly proceeds in a defined orderly manner, but denotes a restraining tendency of one Element upon another. Just as in the Yin-Yang doctrine mutual support and restraint are indispensable, so also the Control cycle functions as a counterbalance to the promotive tendency within the Generative cycle and ensures the maintenance of equilibrium. Classically the Generative cycle is linked to Yin and the Control cycle to Yang. In ancient texts the following symbolism is given to illustrate the ordering of the Control cycle: Wood uproots and loosens Earth; Fire melts Metal; Earth contains and obstructs Water; Metal penetrates and cuts Wood; and Water extinguishes Fire (see illustration 2).

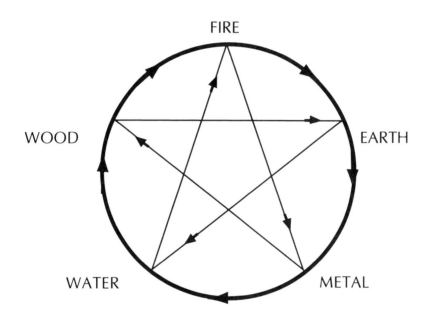

2. The Five Elements:
Generative and Control Cycles

1) Generative cycle follows the outside circle.
2) Control cycle flows within the inner star pattern.

Both these cycles operate simultaneously and unidirectionally creating a natural feedback system. For example, Water controls Fire, but Fire generates Earth which in turn controls Water; by promoting Earth, Fire exerts an indirect counter-influence on Water. The reciprocal relationships among the Elements thus formed, further strengthen the system's tendency towards harmony, though a perniciously excessive or deficient condition in an Element may cause impairment to this self-corrective propensity. In terms of medicine the Five Element philosophy provides a valuable framework in which to describe and understand many aspects of health and illness, particularly the dynamics of the Organs.

The Yin-Yang and Five Element schemes can be partially correlated, for example in the linking of Wood and Fire with Yang since both these Elements are more active as opposed to the more quiescent Yin Elements of Metal and Water, while the Earth sits in neutral balance between Yin and Yang. A selection of traditional correspondences related to the Elements can be viewed in the accompanying chart.

	WOOD	FIRE	EARTH	METAL	WATER
DEVELOPMENT	germination	growth	transformation	maturation	decay/storage
SEASON	spring	summer	late summer*	autumn	winter
DIRECTION	east	south	center	west	north
COLOR	greenish-blue	red	yellow	white	black
PLANET	Jupiter	Mars	Saturn	Venus	Mercury
TASTE	sour	bitter	sweet	pungent	salty
CLIMATIC FACTOR	wind	summer heat	dampness	dryness	cold
YIN ORGAN	Liver	Heart	Spleen	Lung	Kidneys
YANG ORGAN	Gallbladder	Small Intestine	Stomach	Large Intestine	Bladder
SUBSTANCE	Blood	Spirit	Fluids	Qi	Essence
TISSUE	tendon-fascia	blood vessels	muscles	skin/body hair	bones
SENSE ORGAN	eyes	tongue	mouth	nose	ears
EMOTION	anger	jubilance	worry	grief	fear
SOUND	shouting	laughing	melodic	tearful	groaning
VIRTUE	kindness	humility	faithfulness	fairness	wisdom
SECRETION	tears	sweat	saliva	stool/spittle	urine/reproductive
MANIFESTATION	nails	facial color	lips	skin/body hair	teeth/head hair

3. The Five Element Correspondence

* Late summer describes in the Chinese view, the pivot on which the whole year turns; also the Earth may represent the transitional period or pivot between the seasons (usually of 18 days in length).

4
The Essential Substances

Chinese medicine identifies five Substances that form the basis for the development and maintenance of the human body. They are: Qi, Blood (xue), Essence (jing), Spirit (shen) and Fluids (jin ye). The five Substances have a dynamic relationship, supporting and nurturing each other for the benefit of the whole organism. The Substances are also linked with the Elements and Organs according to their special affinities.

Although the classical texts take the concept of Qi for granted, this idea is difficult for the occidental mind to grasp. Qi represents the essential life force within human beings, which is visualized as an internal rarefied substance on the verge of formlessness. Qi as a substance circulates and activates organic functioning, and appears in various differentiated forms. Qi may also be used to denote an actual functioning part of an organism or a particular quality of a phenomenon. Qi is responsible for warming, invigorating and protecting the body, as well as providing orderliness and impetus to its movements and transformations to help ensure integrity.

In the body, Qi is derived from three sources: 1) the Qi, called Original Qi (yuan qi) that is transmitted by the parents at conception, which thereafter determines the basal level of vitality of the body; 2) Grain Qi (gu qi), the nutritionally absorbed energy from foods and liquids; and 3) Cosmic Qi (da qi), the vital portion of the air taken in through respiration.

Basically the body's Qi is differentiated into five major categories:
1) Organ Qi (zang fu qi), which animates all Organs and individualizes an organ's functioning;
2) Meridian Qi (jing qi) is that part of the body's Qi that circulates throughout the comprehensive system of pathways;
3) Nutritive Qi (ying qi) is closely associated with Blood, and aids in he absorption of pure nutrients from digestion and its distribution throughout the whole body;
4) Protective Qi (wei qi) circulates throughout the body (especially superficially); it regulates body temperature and perspiration and warms the Organs;
5) Ancestral Qi (zong qi) aids, regulates and harmonizes respiratory movement and heart beat. Ancestral Qi also motivates the circulation of the Nutritive Qi and Blood.

In Chinese medicine Blood denotes both the material that circulates under the guidance of the heart as well as the force closely associated with the functioning of the sensory organs. The general concept of Blood parallels modern biomedical concepts closely in that its function is to nourish and moisten all the Organs and tissues of the body. The relationship between Blood and Qi is that of Yin to Yang. The Qi is said to be the commander of Blood, while Blood is referred to as the mother of Qi.

Essence determines all human growth and development, as well as the body's physical characteristics. Essence is the foundation of reproductivity, manifesting materially in the form of sperm and ovum and as a force through the procreative urge. Essence is derived from one's parents and is normally produced by the body from the Qi and Blood. The body's Essence matures and is most abundant in adulthood, after puberty. The processes of aging, sexual activity, childbirth and severe prolonged illnesses all lead to a decline in the body's reserve of Essence. Essence is stored in the kidneys and it is distributed from there to the other Organs to form their material basis.

The Spirit is thought to enter the body with the first breath and leave the body with the last. While present in the body, Spirit determines our thoughts, feelings and imaginations, manifesting in both the waking and dream states as consciousness. According to traditional understanding the heart houses the Spirit (i.e. the mind), wherein the integrative functions of consciousness occur, especially during sleep. In contrast, during wakefulness consciousness operates through the brain.

The concept of Spirit in Chinese medicine embraces the occidental notion of mind and soul, although in a more archaic sense. In classical literature Spirit is separated into Yin and Yang aspects referred to as the Animal and Spiritual Soul (po & hun) respectively. The Yin aspect is associated with passion, attachments and instinctual drives with a downward earth-directed movement. After death if the awareness of the Spirit identifies excessively with the Animal Soul due to strong residual earthly attachments, the being may remain as a ghost until placated. Its counterpart, the Yang aspect is associated with imagination, intuition and higher consciousness with an upward, heaven-directed movement. Ideally after death if the Spiritual Soul is totally freed from the Yin Soul's influence, the being attains the mystical soul-body state of an immortal.

The fifth substance, Fluid, is a collective term for all the normal body fluids other than Blood, including saliva, joint, cavity and visceral lubricants, cerebrospinal fluid, sweat, and so on. The Fluids are derived from the ingested food and liquids, and are acted upon by various Organs which spread the Fluids around. The function of the Fluids is to lubricate and moisten all the Organs and tissues throughout the body, including the exterior surfaces of the hair and skin.

5
The Organs

Chinese medicine lays paramount stress on understanding the relationship of the Organs (zang fu) with the various signs and symptoms manifest on the physical, emotional and mental levels of existence. In this way Organs are described in terms of patterns and effects, not in terms of anatomical structure. The term Organ Images (zang xiang) refers to this concept of an Organ's externalization of symptoms via the energetic Meridian system (jing mai). The development of the Organ Image Theory evolved gradually incorporating ancient anatomical knowledge as well as extensive clinical experience. There is evidence that ancient Chinese physicians performed dissection, although the practice fell out of official sanction quickly; thus leaving classical anatomical study incomplete. However much valuable information was nevertheless gathered, including for example the size, weight and placement of major organs, blood vessels and bones, and the heart's role in the circulation of blood. And clinical experience led to the confirmation of many postulated correspondences; as for instance, the observation that healing of a bone fracture is hastened by tonifying the kidneys established a positive relationship between bones and the kidneys.

Chinese medicine in general recognized the functions and patterns of ten Organs (see illustration 4) whose relationships are based upon correspondences with the Yin-Yang and Five Element theories as summarized in the following table:

	YIN ORGAN	YANG ORGAN
WOOD	Liver	Gallbladder
FIRE	Heart	Small Intestine
EARTH	Spleen	Stomach
METAL	Lung	Large Intestine
WATER	Kidneys	Bladder

The Yin-Yang paired Organs of an Element are seen as being connected through certain internal and external Meridians. The Yin Organs are generally more emphasized in Chinese medicine because their functions are closely related to the maintenance of homeostasis both mentally and physically. The Yin Organs in consequence of having a special affinity to the five Substances, absorb, transform, regulate and store them. Yin

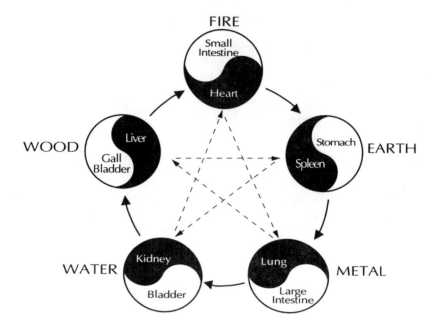

4. The Five Elements

According to the laws of the Five Elements (wu xing) within the body each Element is associated with a Yin and Yang Organ. Also, there exists two important relationships or movements amongst the Elements and Organs. The Generative cycle (represented by the outer circular line) shows what Elements support each other while the Control cycle (inner star pattern) reveals which Elements restrain each other.

Organs are perceived to be more solid and internally placed in the body than Yang Organs, and are possessed of distinctive Nature. Yang Organs, in contrast, are rather hollow and more externally situated within the body cavity, and discharge Substances more than storing them. The Yang Organs deal with the reception, transmission and digestion of food and liquids as well as the elimination of wastes.

The idea of Organ Images relies a great deal on the associations found within the Five Elements. The Organs engender the characteristics of an Element, especially the Yin Organs. For example, the Organs associated with the Wood Element, liver and gallbladder, are easily affected by influences in resonance with that Element, such as the climatic condition of wind, sour food and drinks, the planet Mercury, the color greenish-blue, the season Spring, or the emotion of anger. Disturbances in either Organ project themselves into the body as color changes in the eyes and nails, a possible change in facial color to a greenish-blue hue, a shouting quality in the voice, or emotions such as anger and frustration. Yin-Yang paired Organs are also mutually affected by each other's state of health or disorder. An Organ's Elemental correspondences can be studied by reviewing illustration 3. Listed below are the main functions of the Organs:

1) The liver's primary functions are to control the amount of Blood in circulation and to engender a harmonious, unrestricted flow of Qi throughout the system. A healthy liver facilitates sleeping rhythms, ensures proper vision and allows the emotions to be in appropriate balance.

2) The gallbladder aids the liver and helps in the process of digestion and elimination.

3) The heart's function is to circulate the Blood and control the Blood Vessels, as well as to regulate the mind.

4) Classically the small intestine is said to separate the pure from the impure, converting food and liquids into nutrition and passing on the wastes.

5) The spleen functions are to alchemically transform nutrients and produce Blood, to regulate the amount of Fluids in circulation and to prevent Blood from hemorrhaging. Additionally the spleen sustains the flow of Qi against gravity so that Nutrient-Blood reaches the lung and heart and the abdominal Organs are kept in their proper elevated position.

6) The stomach's main function is to receive and break down food and liquids, then pass on the absorbed nutrients to the spleen for further transformation. The stomach also assumes the role of causing Qi to descend downward to guarantee that its contents are passed along the Intestines for further processing and elimination.

7) The lung draws in Cosmic Qi and through its harmonious rhythmic movement disperses the Qi throughout the body and especially down to the kidneys. In addition, since Qi leads the Fluids, the lung is in charge of dispersing Fluids.

8) The large intestine is responsible for the elimination and discharge of the body's solid wastes.

9) The kidneys are generally considered to be the root of the physical body, storing and transmuting Essence. The kidneys also produce marrow, which is of two types: bone and spinal. Thus the kidneys influence the vibrancy of mental functioning, since the physical brain is considered a part of the spinal marrow. The kidneys also control the reproductive organs and secretions. They regulate the balance of Fluids, sending turbid liquids downwards and re-cycling clear Fluids back into general circulation. Furthermore the kidneys grasp the Qi and thereby assist the lung in directing the Qi downward. Finally the kidneys perform the function of storing the Original Qi.

10) The bladder temporarily stores and then discharges the turbid liquid wastes in harmony with the kidneys.

Apart from the above mentioned ten major Organs and their associated Meridians, Chinese medicine also recognizes the Triple Burner (san jiao) and the Heart Protector (xin bao), neither of which are Organs in the usual sense. The *Classic of Difficult Issues* says that the Heart Protector and the Triple Burner represent inside and outside, both having a name but no form. The concept of 'no form' is to be understood in two ways, literally in the sense of not having a defined structure, and in the Taoist sense as denoting a charged precursor state of manifestation (like the cosmic, primordial Void) of a phenomenon. Though both Organs are more akin to energy fields than to structures, they too have specific external Meridians associated with them; hence one speaks of twelve Meridians.

The Triple Burner originates out of the "moving Qi between the kidneys", which is another name for the Original Qi found below the umbilicus. The Triple Burner divides itself into distinct fields: a) Upper Burner (above the diaphragm); b) Middle Burner (between the navel and the diaphragm); and c) Lower Burner (below the navel).

The Triple Burner's main function is to transmit the Original Qi. The kidneys store the Original Qi while the Triple Burner helps distribute it to the other Organs and throughout the body. Also the Triple Burner assists in circulating the Ancestral, Nutritive and the Defensive Qi which are centered and issue forth from the Upper, Middle and Lower Burners, respectively.

Both Triple Burner and kidneys have an influence on the body's regulation of heat through their connection to the Original Qi that forms the body's basal energy level. Triple Burner also assists the circulation of Defensive Qi that warms and protects the body. From this perspective, and considering that the kidneys are the only organs situated retroperitoneal (behind the abdominal lining), the Triple Burner may function through the fascial linings of the peritoneum and pleura to energetically insulate and protect the Organs.

The Heart Protector is located within the chest, acting as a buffer to protect the heart, physically and psychologically. Just as the Triple Burner may energetically function through abdominal fascial linings, the Heart Protector may utilize the pericardium as its medium. Though there has been an endless debate as to the correspondence of the Heart Protector and Triple Burner to the Five Elements, they clearly appear to have a harmonizing and mediating role and are of great clinical significance.

Other organs such as the brain, bones, womb and the blood vessels, though recognized by Chinese medicine, are formulated to exist independently of any external Meridian. Yet other organs and glands found in modern medicine such as the thyroid, pancreas and adrenals are not distinguished by Chinese medicine; however, their functions do appear under the various Organ Images.

6
The Meridian System

*T*he concept and practical use of the Meridian System distinguishes Chinese medicine from other ancient healing traditions. The *Inner Classic* states: "The Meridians move the Qi and Blood, regulate the Yin and the Yang, moisten the tendons and the Bones, and benefit the joints . . . internally the Meridians connect with the Organs and externally with the joints, limbs and the outer surface of the body." The ancient Chinese perceived that within the body there exists a whole network of subtle three-dimensional pathways linking and balancing the various structures, Substances, Organs and spheres of influence.

The Meridian System has specifically four major functions:

1) To promote communication between the internal Organs and the exterior of the body, and to connect the individual to the rhythms of the biosphere and the celestial energies. 2) To regulate and harmonize the Yin and Yang as seen in the activities of the Organs and Substances. 3) To distribute Qi from the Organs to the body. 4) To protect the body by creating a protective shield.

There are seven different types of pathways referred to in the theory of the Meridian System. Of these, the twelve Regular Meridians (zheng jing) and the eight Extraordinary Vessels (ba mai) are of principal importance. The other five types of pathways are of lesser importance and act primarily as supports and extensions to the Regular Meridians and Extraordinary Vessels.

The twelve Regular Meridians connect internally to the Organs and externally to the surface of the skin. Each Meridian is distributed bilaterally and symmetrically on the body, being named after its respective associated Organ. The twelve Meridians are divided equally into Yin or Yang groups according to their pertinent Organ's classification and are subdivided by their distribution to either the hand or the foot. Generally if you imagine a person standing with the hands above the head, the Qi within the Yin Meridians flows from the ground upward (i.e. from foot to chest to hand); while in the Yang Meridians, Qi flows from ceiling downward (i.e. from hand to head to foot) (see illustration 5).

The Qi of the twelve Regular Meridians travels in a fixed direction, each Meridian transferring its Qi to the next Meridian where they meet. Yin Meridians meet in the chest, Yang Meridians meet in the head, and

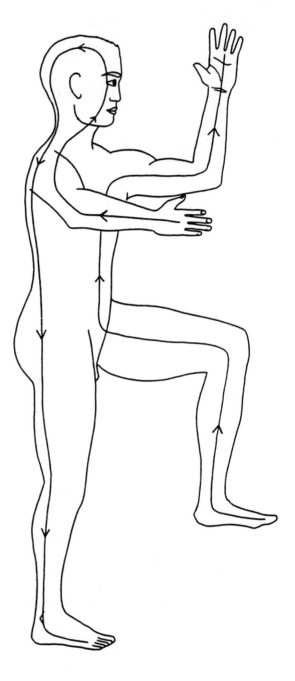

Qi of Yin Meridians
flow upward

Qi of Yang Meridians
flow downward

5. Meridian Qi Flow

both Yin and Yang Meridians conjoin at the distal ends of the extremities. This fixed directional flow takes a complete day to make one cycle and is synchronized with the ancient Chinese twelve hour day. According to this diurnal concept of the Meridian flow, which is fundamentally an ancient codification of the body's subtle biological (circadian) rhythms, each Organ and thus its Meridian achieves its peak level of vitality during an allocated hour (a roughly two-hour period in our time reckoning), the whole cycle beginning and ending at 3 am, at the junction of liver and lung.

When an excess or deficient condition within an Organ or Meridian exists, symptoms may manifest during its specific hour within the daily cycle. Usually these are the recurring symptoms often found in chronic disorders; for example, patients with liver imbalance often wake up out of deep sleep between 1 and 3 am and have difficulty returning to sleep. The following is a list of time relationships within the Organ-Meridian Qi flow:

HOUR	ORGAN-MERIDIAN
3am–5am	Lung
5am–7am	Large Intestine
7am–9am	Stomach
9am–11am	Spleen
11am–1pm	Heart
1pm–3pm	Small Intestine
3pm–5pm	Bladder
5pm–7pm	Kidneys
7pm–9pm	Heart Protector
9pm–11pm	Triple Burner
11pm–1am	Gallbladder
1am–3am	Liver

In comparison, the eight Extraordinary Vessels function as reservoirs for the Regular Meridians, supplementing or storing the Qi of the Meridians as needed, contributing in this way to the overall balance within the Meridian System. While the Regular Meridians are perceived as subtle thread- like pathways, the Vessels are considered broad receptacles for the Qi. Furthermore, the Extraordinary Vessels are considered a primary force in embryological development, being responsible for the organization of the embryonic terrain and early life's structural development. Of the eight Extraordinary Vessels, the Conception (ren), Governing (du) and Penetrating (chong) Vessels originate first.

The Governing Vessel is named after its function of regulating the Yang Meridians by acting as their reservoir. The Conception Vessel regulates the Yin Meridians and is so named because its external pathway corresponds to the linea nigra, the dark line that appears on the abdomen during pregnancy. The Penetrating Vessel is said to regulate the twelve Regular Meridians and Blood, being so named after its deep pathway. Also of importance is the Belt Vessel which, along with the above three core Vessels, forms the nucleus of the embryonic formative force.

The other four Vessels, known as the Yin and Yang Heel (qiao) Vessels and the Yin and Yang Linking (wei) Vessels, are of secondary manifestation and significance, functioning to protect, restrain and counterbalance the outward moving tendency of the three core Vessels. These four secondary Vessels also provide reservoir functions for the Regular Meridians.

Along the Regular Meridians and the Conception and Governing Vessels there exist a number of Qi holes or points (xue) where the energetic influences found within the pathway become concentrated and accessible to manipulation through certain therapeutic techniques such as acupuncture and massage, or for use in diagnosis. The six other Vessels do not have independent points along their external projections but share points found along the Regular Meridians (see illustration 6).

Archaeology offers evidence that there was a progressive evolution within the Meridian System theory. The most ancient manuscripts to date that mention the Meridians are scrolls that pre-date China's first medical canon, the *Inner Classic*, by about two centuries. These scrolls, which were recently unearthed in the Mawangdui tombs, mention the practice of moxibustion, and specify eleven Meridians whose names and trajectories in the body differ from those currently accepted today. Nor do the Mawangdui manuscripts suggest any mutual interconnection between the meridians. Puncturing the body with stone needles was documented in various texts as far back as the 8th century B.C., but the *Inner Classic* holds the view that the practices of acupuncture and moxibustion arose separately. In fact, acupuncture is said to have come from the east, where it was utilized to combat disorders that arose from the frequent winds of that region, while moxibustion originated in the north (probably Mongolia) where people used it to treat conditions that developed from cold influences. By the time of the *Inner Classic*, however, these two modalities were already integrated into a single system.

History suggests that the knowledge and use of these concentration points preceded the development of the Meridian theory, for stone needling was practiced even in the ancient times. In old China the idea of the existence of influential points on the body was akin to the idea of influential points on the earth in the science of geomancy (feng shui). Geomancy was the traditional science used to determine appropriate auspicious sites for such tasks as the burial of the dead or the building of a temple. Geomancy was also used as an art of divination. Many of the concentration point names (for a numbering system was not used until quite recently) still reflect this connection to certain landscape themes, such as rivers, hills, pools and mounds. Other point names display astrological, anatomical, animal or functional motifs.

Each concentration point has its own unique therapeutic properties and characteristics. In course of time it was discovered that certain point patterns and groupings shared common properties and were linked internally to specific Organs. Undoubtedly, the meditative practices and insights of the sages and extensive clinical research by the ancient doctors provided a fertile ground for the energetic mapping of the body. In consequence of these diverse inquiries, besides numerous separate points with their individual properties, a total of 361 common concentration points on the Meridians and Vessels were recognized.

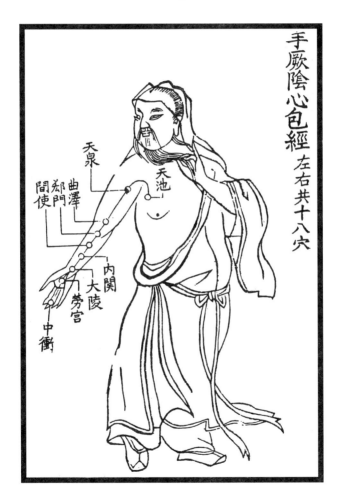

6. Classical Meridian Drawing

A classical Chinese medical drawing of the Heart Protector Meridian (xin baojing) and its nine Qi holes or points (xue). This meridian's external route starts from the chest and moves down the inside of the arm to the middle finger.

7
Disease Causation

Pathogenic forces disturb the body's equilibrium and harmony with the surrounding environment. In Chinese medicine, illnesses are classified according to whether they originate from an internal or external cause. Once this equilibrium is lost, disease patterns become entrenched and develop according to an intrinsic progression. Internally, the delicate metabolic balancing process is usually disrupted by imbalanced emotions or lifestyle habits.

External factors that cause illness arise generally from two sources: a) climatic disorders related to excessive or prolonged exposure to one of the six exogenous Pernicious Influences (liu yin): wind, summer heat, dampness, dryness, cold and fire; b) pestilential substances in a variety of forms. The theory of pestilential substances, developed during the Ming Dynasty (1368-1644 A.D.) concerns contagious diseases that are transmitted through nose and mouth. Specific patterns are associated with each pestilence, and this idea parallels the modern concept of infectious pathogens.

The six Pernicious Influences are individually named after the normal climatic condition of a season that often leads to its formation. For example the over-exposure to cold that usually occurs in winter can progress into a pathogenic cold pattern in the body if resistance and adaptability are weak. Each Pernicious Influence is also associated with Yin or Yang according to its effect; a Yin excess injures the body's Yang and a Yang excess injures the body's Yin. Wind, summerheat, dryness and fire are Yang forms of excess; while dampness and cold are classified as Yin. The affinities between the seasons and Organs with excess patterns follow the Five Element theory.

In Chinese medicine the symptoms that a Pernicious Influence produces, mimic the characteristics of its corresponding prototype in the environment. This is summarized as follows: summerheat and fire both are characterized by an increase of temperature (summerheat is specifically related to the summer season, while fire is non-specific to a particular season); cold by a decrease in temperature; dampness is distinguished by an increased presence of water; dryness by a decreased presence of water; and wind by a tendency for abruptness and changeability.

The individual Pernicious Influences initially enter the body through the skin or respiratory system, and then penetrate via the Meridians into the Organs. These influences may invade the body individually or in combination (such as Damp and Heat together). Once a climatic excess lodges itself within the body, it may transform itself into another excess pattern; for example, a cold pattern may turn into heat after some time. Generally, the body is most vulnerable to Pernicious Influences during the transitions between the seasons if the body's natural ability to self-regulate and remain harmonious with the surrounding environment is deficient.

The names and characteristics of the six exogenous Pernicious Influences are also used to describe internal Organ induced excesses. When a deficiency of either Yin, Yang, Qi or other Substance occurs in one of the Organs, this may produce an endogenous Pernicious Influence often associated with their Five Element affinity (refer to illustration # 3). For example, when the Yin aspect of the liver becomes deficient, the liver may generate endogenous Wind excess.

For the disorders originating internally the emotions are of paramount importance. Emotional responsiveness is considered healthy and is to a large extent socially and parentally conditioned. Specific emotions according to Chinese medicine are seen as extensions of, or resonations with the Qi of an Organ. Under circumstances such as blocked emotional expression or abrupt, intense or prolonged emotional stimulation, all of which exceed the capacity of the individual to self-regulate, illness starts. The mechanism of imbalance due to the emotions occurs through their effect on the flow of Qi as stated in the *Inner Classic*: "Anger causes the Qi to flow upwards; excessive jubilance scatters and slows the Qi; sadness and grief weakens the Qi; fear causes the Qi to descend; fright drives the Qi into disorder; and worry makes the Qi stagnate."

These changes in the flow of Qi not only hamper the circulation of other Substances but also resonate with a specific Organ's Qi according to their Five Element correspondence. For example, prolonged worry will cause the Qi to stagnate. This directly affects the spleen's function of transforming food and liquids, thus resulting in a symptomatic pattern of indigestion, abdominal distension and pain, and may be instrumental in the eventual formation of gastro-intestinal ulcers. Furthermore, according to Chinese circular thinking, a prolonged physical or functional imbalance within an Organ can further create a receptivity towards certain emotions; for example liver Qi stagnation could lead to depression, difficulty in expressing frustrations and still later to angry outbursts.

Additionally, the malfunctioning body can produce two pathological auto-toxins: Phlegm (tan) and Stagnant Blood (yu xue). These may appear in various organs or parts of the body and in turn generate other disorders. Phlegm originates from a disturbance of water metabolism most often associated with faulty digestion, and wherein body fluids turn morbid and condense. Phlegm produces a wide variety of symptoms, easily causes obstructions and can even generate lumps and other hard swellings such as tumors. Thus it may be seen that Phlegm in Chinese medicine has a broader meaning which is not confined to sputum alone.

Stagnant Blood is caused by a number of factors: trauma or hemorrhaging may injure the Blood causing it to coagulate. Once Stagnant Blood forms, the flow of Qi and Blood through that area becomes impeded and the local tissues remain unnourished, since Stagnant Blood is devitalized. Stagnant Blood appears in fixed places and produces pain and swelling.

Lifestyle, especially diet, sexual and physical activity and disturbances of the natural rhythms of life, plays an important role in causing illness. Traditionally each type of food and liquid according to its taste (corresponding to the Elements) and temperature (i.e. whether heating or cooling to the body) is considered to affect specific Organs or Substances. Consumption of spoiled food, or overindulgence of a particular taste or temperature of foods are to be avoided lest they aggravate an Organ or cause susceptibility to a climatic Pernicious Influence. The meals should preserve the balance of tastes and temperatures, and should ideally be partaken in moderate quantities at regular times. Moderation, regularity and the avoidance of extremes is also recommended in the traditional view for sexuality and physical activity in China, so that the Organs and Substances would not be harmed. Overall living in accord with the laws of nature and to remain in tune with the seasons and celestial forces was seen as the essence of preventative medicine.

The progression of disease after its onset and during its course is analyzed in light of two opposing forces: the strength of the anti-pathogenic component, that is, the body's defensive capability and self-healing mechanism as a reflection of the vitality of the body's Qi; and the vigor of the pathogenic influences. The struggle between these two forces follows the laws of Yin-Yang producing as a result either excess or deficiency. Generally in deficient type patterns the anti-pathogenic force (i.e. the body's Qi) is impaired while in excess patterns the pathogenic factors predominate. In either case the anti-pathogenic forces must prevail for the Yin-Yang balance to be restored to normal, and to regain health. If this is not achieved, the process of a downward spiral with a progressive weakening of the energetic, physiological and physical structure and increased severity of symptoms ultimately leading to a premature termination of life, will have commenced.

8
Diagnosis and Differentiation

*T*he intent of Chinese medical examination is to elucidate the origin, location and nature of the patient's illness. The task then shifts to organizing and differentiating the information gathered through the examination so that an appropriate treatment may be prescribed. According to the concept of human integrity in Chinese medicine, a doctor can comprehend the totality of a patient's imbalance through careful examination because of the body's innate wholeness. For example, the interior and exterior aspects of the body are considered to be functionally interconnected with and responsive to one another, and so whenever an internal disease arises it will also manifest some form of disturbance on or near the body's surface. Likewise, general conditions, such as chronic fatigue, are connected with and form the basis of specific conditions, such as acute headache. Therefore, general and specific, and chronic and acute conditions are considered interdependent.

Classically there are four examinations: visual observation, listening-smelling, palpation and inquiry. In the visual method of diagnosis the examination concentrates on the appearance of the person as regards to physique, expression and complexion. Furthermore, physical changes of the sensory orifices are noted along with any abnormal secretions or excretions. Finally and of great clinical importance: the tongue is examined for its mobility, shape, color and coating. The tongue reflects the state of the Organs, Substances and the presence of any Pernicious Influences with great accuracy. The clinical examination of the tongue and pulse are the two preeminent methods of diagnosis in Chinese medicine.

The listening-smelling method (these words are conjoined because the Chinese character denotes both activities) places attention on the quality and strength of the voice; the rhythm, strength and depth of the breathing and abnormal sounds and odors exuded by the body.

The inquiry part of the examination shifts to the subjective nature of the illness. Usually questions can cover a wide territory from food preferences and emotions to the regularity of bowel movements. The following is a condensed traditional list of topics of inquiry: sensations of heat or coldness; perspiration; pains or unusual sensations; appetite and thirst; the elimination of wastes; sleep; one's daily routine; previous health history; reproductive problems and cycles; and the onset and development of the present illness. The specific questions asked are guided by the nature of the disorder and the initial impressions derived from other methods of diagnosis.

Finally, in palpation, the Meridians, points and the tissues are felt to ascertain important information about the nature of the illness. The abdomen is also palpated, the Japanese having particularly refined abdominal diagnosis. Special emphasis is placed on feeling the wrist pulse, for here a global impression of the body can be perceived along with specific information about the Organs and Meridians. The wrist pulse is divided into three positions and at each position a pair of Yin-Yang Organs of the same Element can be felt in the deep and superficial location (see illustration 7).

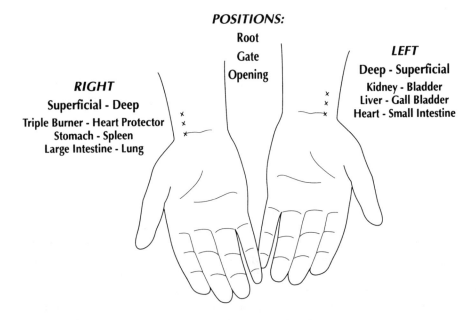

POSITIONS:
Root
Gate
Opening

LEFT
Deep - Superficial
Kidney - Bladder
Liver - Gall Bladder
Heart - Small Intestine

RIGHT
Superficial - Deep
Triple Burner - Heart Protector
Stomach - Spleen
Large Intestine - Lung

7. Chinese Pulse Positions
(the right and left root position are also said to reflect
the kidney yang and yin respectively.)

At different Organ positions the strength, depth, smoothness, rhythm, frequency and amplitude of the pulses is carefully noted and classified according to one or more combinations of the classical twenty-eight types. The art of pulse diagnosis is a refined practice that requires good clinical instruction, sensitivity and extensive experience to master but is worth the investment of time and energy in its study because of the invaluable information it reveals. Patients in Asian countries often judge a traditional doctor's expertise by his or her level of pulse mastery, as evidenced by the accuracy with which the doctor interprets and recites their symptoms by feeling the pulse alone.

Once the four examinations are complete the practitioner differentiates the information into recognizable patterns. According to different historical schools of Chinese medical thought, various ways to categorize and organize patterns emerged. The most important patterning models are the Eight Guiding Principles (ba gang), followed by differentiation according to Substance, Organ manifestation, Meridian and causative factor. All these models are further understood and integrated with the correspondences outlined in the theory of the Five Elements. Each pattern describes the body in its present functioning state and denotes which stage an illness is in. Thus patterns change as the person moves towards or away from balance. This requires the frequent reassessment of the patient's situation in anticipation of change from one pattern to another in the course of a disorder.

Typically the Eight Guiding Principles are used first to classify the signs and symptoms and define the parameters of the illness. These Principles consist of four pairs of opposites: Yin and Yang, interior and exterior, cold and heat, and deficiency and excess. Specifically Yin-Yang are used to denote the general character of an illness; interior-exterior describes the depth of disease activity in the body; cold-heat describes the specific thermal nature of disease; while deficiency-excess describes the state of the body's Qi versus the pathogenic forces within the body. In actuality the four pairs of opposites are subdivisions of the primary Yin-Yang pair and help define the strength, quality and location of the disease. Following this categorization the clinician uses other pattern models to further differentiate and guide in the selection of the most appropriate therapy.

Substance patterns relate to the condition of the five fundamental Substances. The Qi, Blood and Fluids are usually classified according to deficiency, stagnation or directionally inappropriate flow, while Essence and Spirit usually only manifest deficient patterns. Organ patterns relate mostly to the deficient or excess state of Yin and Yang, Qi and sometimes Blood aspects within an Organ, or if there is an endogenous Pernicious Influence present. The Meridian patterns relate to the presence of distinctive symptoms found along the course of a Meridian or Vessel pathway, independent of an Organ's disharmony. Another patterning model, the Six Stages (liu jing bing), is frequently used in Internal Medicine. The Six Stages is useful for assessing the depth of penetration and severity of a Pernicious Influence (especially cold) through the Meridian system. Patterns relating to a causative factor include primarily the six exogenous Pernicious Influences and emotions as well as specific patterns due to Phlegm, Stagnant Blood, Pestilence, traumatic injuries etc.

Distinct diseases are noted in Chinese medicine, such as diabetes, depression or parasitic infestation. First however, each of these distinctive diseases is differentiated according to the above mentioned pattern models to determine the individual's response to that disease process before a treatment strategy is instituted. In reverse, many times different specific diseases may be treated by a common approach because they share a common pattern at their root; for example liver Qi stagnation may be the cause of goiter, irregular menstruation, depression or abdominal pain. Thus an important principle in Chinese medicine is to treat different diseases by the same methods and to apply different methods to the same disease, according to need.

In addition to the above models for pattern categorization there is the less commonly used approach of analyzing and treating constitutional types based upon Yin-Yang and/or Five Element correspondence. In this mode of assessment both the physical characteristics and emotional-mental traits are differentiated. The value of this approach is in preventative therapy and in understanding the configuration of signs and symptoms in chronic illness by viewing the person's situation from its long-term perspective. As in all patterning systems of Chinese medicine the focus is on the person, whether one uses the constitutional approach or the more "here and now" patterning models.

9
Therapeutic Modalities and Ideas

*T*here are five basic methods leading to the restoration of health that are essential to the practitioner's understanding. According to the *Inner Classic*: the first method is to cure the Spirit, the second gives knowledge on how to nourish the body, the third teaches the efficaciousness of medicines, the fourth elucidates the use of acupuncture-moxibustion, and the fifth gives instruction on the examination of the Organs, Qi and Blood. These therapeutic principles are described in the *Inner Classic* as having developed in a sequential order over time to address the ever-deteriorating level of health in society.

The *Inner Classic* teaches that in the ancient past the sages guided the members of the community towards a harmonious life in accord with the Tao. The *Inner Classic* describes life in that ideal age as follows- "The men in antiquity lived among their animals. They pursued a vigorous and active life, avoiding in this manner the effects of cold. They sought out the shade, thereby avoiding the effects of heat. Their inner life knew no exhaustion from emotions and their external life was without interference from others. In that peaceful world evil was unable to penetrate deeply into the body. Potent drugs were unnecessary for internal treatment and acupuncture inappropriate for external therapy. Instead, it was sufficient to invoke the gods and effect cure through the assimilation of refined essences." Therefore, the invocation of the gods and self-cultivation was considered sufficient to heal the mild disorders present in that age. The *Inner Classic* further describes that when human beings lost their original naturalness, and humanity became increasingly violent and selfish, more complex disorders arose leading to the necessity for progressively stronger forms of therapy. Finally, systematic forms of diagnosis and medical theory had to be developed in order to properly comprehend illness and to categorize knowledge of healing for the benefit of subsequent generations.

Accompanying this systemization of medicine certain principles of treatment were refined and organized. Paramount among these principles is the concept of Root and Branch (bao ben tong zhi). The Root refers to the primary cause and symptoms of a disease as well as to the state of the body's resistance. The Branch refers to the general nature and secondary symptoms of the disease as also to the state of the pathogenic factors involved.

In clinical practice this treatment model is helpful in ascertaining whether the Root or the Branch should be treated first. In acute manifestations of illness, generally the Branch would be treated first, and once the more severe symptoms have abated will then be followed by Root treatment. In chronic cases however, the Root, the underlying cause, needs to be diagnosed and treated, often in disregard of the Branch to effectuate a thorough restoration of the whole person. But for chronic situations where symptoms are severe and painful, a combined strategy of treating Root and Branch concurrently is essential. In critical circumstances during the course of a chronic illness, palliative treatment of the Branch is the first necessity, while the Root is not addressed initially so as to forego taxing the delicate vitality of the patient.

Another important principle of treatment is that of Yin-Yang reconciliation, i.e. to reduce conditions of excess and to build up conditions of deficiency. In practice usually this is done directly to the Organ, Meridian, Substance or to the pathogenic factor present.

In all situations, once there is a positive progression towards balance, attention will once again shift to prevention by strengthening the body's ability to self-regulate and adapt to its environment; thereby avoiding future maladies. This philosophy is expressed in a Chinese proverb: "Waiting to treat illness after they manifest is like waiting to dig a well after one is thirsty."

In Chinese medical therapy acupuncture-moxibustion, Internal Medicine (therapeutic use of medicinal substances), dietetics, massage and remedial exercises are utilized as the principle modalities. All these modalities share a common theoretical foundation and if required, can be applied in combination. Surgery is used sometimes when all else fails. The venerated physician Hua Tuo who lived in the Eastern Han Dynasty (25-220 A.D.) is credited for his great surgical skill and promoted the use of Indian hemp anesthesia. It was unfortunate, however, that after the era of Hua Tuo, surgery was largely neglected until modern times.

Diet and the usage of medicinal substances from plant, animal and mineral kingdoms depended upon the organizational models of Yin-Yang and the Five Element theories. Specifically, substances were classified by temperature, i.e. cold, cool, warm and hot; by taste, which is broken down into sour, bitter, sweet, pungent and salty; by direction of action, which indicates whether the substance has an ascending, descending, floating or sinking tendency; and by the Organ and Meridian they affect.

In Internal Medicine and pharmacology the four divisions of a medicinal substance's temperature relate to the thermal effect it has upon the body. For example, skullcap root and chrysanthemum flowers are known to be cold in nature and therefore useful in treating fevers; while cinnamon bark and ginger root being hot, warm the body when chilled. In terms of Yin and Yang theory the hot and warm temperatures are Yang in nature, while cold and cool temperatures are Yin.

The five tastes are each representative of one of the Five Elements as follows, Wood:sour, Fire:bitter, Earth:sweet, Metal:pungent and Water:salty. In addition, some substances are classified as being bland or lacking in flavor. These are grouped with the sweet taste. In general sweet, bland and pungent are considered to be Yang in effect; while sour, bitter and salty have a Yin effect. Specifically the tastes are associated with certain actions and effects on the Qi.

Sourness has an astringent action; it arrests discharge, promotes digestion and has an overall concentrating effect on the Qi. Hawthorne berries and lemons are examples of plants with a sour taste.

Bitterness is considered to be eliminative, anti-inflammatory and detoxifying in action, with the effect of discharging Qi downward. Mugwort leaves, rhubarb root and cascara bark may be cited as examples of bitter taste.

Sweetness and those substances that are bland in taste have a nourishing, harmonizing and tonic action, while tending to slow down the flow of Qi. Licorice root and dates are predominately of the sweet taste.

Pungency or spiciness have both a stimulating and dispersing action that raises and quickens the pace of Qi. Ginger root, prepared aconite root and peppers are noted for their pungent taste.

Saltiness has a softening and moistening action, with the effect of dissolving Qi that has become congealed as, for example, in hard abdominal masses. Most forms of seaweed typically possess a salty taste.

To understand a substance comprehensively both temperature and taste must be taken into account together. For example, if two plants are both hot but possess different flavors (such as pungent and bitter), their actions will be different in the body. Also substances are recognized to have particular affinities to certain specific Organs and Meridians; these associations are usually derived from empirical experience.

Generally the direction of action is in harmony with a substance's taste and temperature according to their relationship with Yin or Yang. This is summarized below:

	YANG	YIN
DIRECTION	Ascending-Floating	Descending-Sinking
TEMPERATURE	Hot-Warm	Cold-Cool
TASTE	Pungent-Sweet-Bland	Sour-Bitter-Salty

The ascending and descending tendencies refer explicitly to a substance's effect on redirecting the Qi either upwards or downwards. Floating has the main effect of dispersing the Qi outward to dispel external Pernicious Influences. Sinking has a concentrating effect on the Qi, moving it inward and downwards; this being specifically useful in promoting mental tranquillity. In the most general sense, substances are used therapeutically to counteract the nature of the illness. Thus Yin symptom patterns are treated with substances that have a Yang taste, temperature and direction of action, and vice versa for Yang diseases.

Historically the configuration of a plant or mineral has also been used in Chinese medicine to determine its appropriate use. Configuration refers to shape, texture, color, moisture and its natural environmental origins. A good example of this concept is the ginseng root that is shaped similar to the human body, with head, arms and legs. This plant is native to cold, mountainous regions of north China and Korea. It has a long growth cycle that takes about 7 years to reach maturity. Ginseng is said to be an excellent tonic that nourishes and warms the whole body, and also promotes longevity. In fact, the Chinese characters for ginseng (or ren shen in pinyin) literally mean "man root".

A unique feature of Internal Medicine is the highly evolved art of formulation. A physician is not only required to know the individual substances, but also the strategies of treatment and most importantly the complex ways in which medicinal substances combine and interact therapeutically. Specifically there are 8 general strategies of treatment and around 20 types of formula categories to select from.

The traditional strategies of treatment in Internal Medicine include: sweating, vomiting, clearing, draining, harmonizing, warming, reducing, and tonifying. Each strategy focuses on different key causes to ill health, principally: sweating is utilized to dispel invading Pernicious Influences; vomiting is effective in excess toxic conditions in the upper digestive tract; clearing refers to loosening and de-congesting the Blood, Qi or Fluids; draining is useful to purge the large intestine of accumulation; harmonizing denotes restoring balance amongst the malfunctioning Organs; warming dispels coldness and strengthens the Yang; reducing refers to lowering the body's temperature when there is excess heat; and lastly, tonifying is used to build up the deficient conditions of Yin, Yang, Blood or Qi.

The formula categories are extensions of these treatment strategies and broadly organize the formulas according to their clinical presentation. Each formula or prescription will normally contain four classes of ingredients arranged in a hierarchical fashion, being referred to as the chief, deputy, assistant and envoy. The chief is the principal ingredient, specific to the patient's pattern or illness and thus indispensable to the formula. The deputy either acts to strengthen the principal ingredient's effect or serves as the main ingredient directed against a co-existing pattern. The assistant helps to reinforce the effect of the chief and deputy ingredients or treats secondary manifestations of the disease pattern, or contains ingredients that check the toxic side effects of the other ingredients in the formula. The envoy directs the above to their appropriate site and/or harmonizes the various actions of the other ingredients.

Not all formulas contain the full hierarchy of ingredients, while others contain a number of ingredients in each class within the hierarchy. There are hundreds of formulas of both classical and modern origins in use today. Ideally each formula is tailored to meet the needs of a particular patient's condition, although pre-made standardized formulas are now readily available. These combinations of medicines have a synergetic effect that is different from the sum total of its ingredients. The medicines are administered in a wide variety of forms: decoction, pills, powders, plasters, medicinal wines and syrups.

Acupuncture and massage therapy are considered more of a Yang, external form of therapy. The focus of these therapies is to remove blockages (especially of Qi) in the Meridian System so that Yin-Yang, Substances and Organs can communicate and function harmoniously. This idea is expressed in the axiom found in the *Inner Classic*: "Where there is communication there is no pain; where there is pain, communication is obstructed." "Pain" here includes both somatic and emotional suffering. Acupuncture is not only effective for painful syndromes, but also for all sort of illnesses like chronic indigestion or gastrointestinal ulcers; menstrual problems; musculoskeletal complaints such as lower back pain and tendinitis; mental depression and emotional disorders; hearing loss; asthma; viral illnesses, such as chronic fatigue syndrome and viral hepatitis; and so on.

Acupuncture is the method of applying delicate thin needles to pierce the body at specific points. These needles were made classically of various metals depending on their intended effect; gold, for example, has a tonifying effect, while silver tends to sedate. In modern times more durable stainless steel needles, which have a neutral effect, are most commonly used. The effect of needling is also determined by the method of insertion and manipulation once in place, the breathing sequence of the patient, the intention of the practitioner, as well as the specific therapeutic qualities of the Meridian and point selected. Needless to say, acupuncture is a precise technical science as well as an art that requires a great deal of skill and experience to master.

Moxibustion is an application of heat to the chosen focal point. Mugwort (artemisia vulgaris) is the herb of choice, even though others are also used. A small portion of the dried ignited herb is placed on the skin directly or held slightly above the surface. The patient feels warmth at the focal point, and in cases where necessary the skin may sometimes be cauterized producing a powerful effect to stimulate the flow of Qi and to tonify the body's Yang. Other adjunctive techniques such as micro-bloodletting on the acupuncture points, or cupping—a type of localized suction technique, may also be used under special conditions.

Interestingly, the written form of the term for Chinese medicine, "zhong yi", is composed of two characters, the first is "zhong" 中 meaning middle, as in the Middle Kingdom, what we call China. The second character "yi" 醫 standing for medicine is, however, again composed of two, a root and a phonetic character. The root character "yu" 酉 shows a jar which is used for keeping fermented liquors (which could be medicinal wines or cordials). The phonetic character "yi" 殹 means to take out arrows "shu" 殳 from the quiver "yi" 医, referring to the practice of acupuncture and possibly ancient sorcery (killing the demons that cause disease). The written expression for "medicine" thus reflects the nature of the therapeutic approaches that medicine embraces.

Therapeutic massage is widely practiced for all manner of illnesses, and is especially preferred over acupuncture for treating children. Techniques of massage include manually activating the points and Meridians, kneading and rubbing the soft tissues, manipulating the joints, bonesetting and massaging the viscera. In the field of remedial exercise both ritualized calisthenics and breathing techniques such as Qi Gong and Tai Qi Quan are used to promote self-healing and to prevent disease.

In the modern era many impressive new procedures have been developed, some in conjunction with modern medicine, such as acupuncture anesthesia, which is useful in some types of surgery. New medicines using a combination of western and oriental pharmaceutical substances and techniques have also been introduced. Another important development has been the theory and practice of various acupuncture microsystems. One such is auricular acupuncture, through which the whole body can be treated via the ear alone. Qi Gong, a method of directing the Qi in the body via the breath, has also grown popular for self-healing in conditions such as cancer, arthritis and chronic painful disorders.

Often a practitioner specializes in one field of therapeutics, like acupuncture or massage, or in a branch of medicine, such as pediatrics or gynecology. Nevertheless, the higher vision of educating and inspiring everyone to live in harmony with nature has always been an important goal of Chinese medical practitioners.

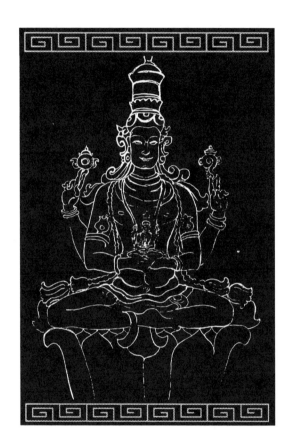

PART TWO
AYURVEDA

1
Origins and Development

*T*he word "Ayurveda," which comes from the Vedas, the ancient sacred books of the Aryans, means "the Lore of Life." Ayurveda, whose origins go back at least five thousand years, began as an appendix to the youngest of the Vedas, the *Atharva Veda*. Most of the Vedic healing lore occurs in the *Atharva Veda*, which is basically a manual of magic (see illustration 8). After its incantational medicine evolved into empirical medicine, the most important of all Ayurvedic texts, the *Charaka Samhita*, appeared, possibly between the 8th and 10th centuries B.C. Ayurveda's most famous surgical text, the *Sushruta Samhita*, was also compiled around this time. While these texts may have had single authors they are more likely to be compilations of material from many sources.

Ayurvedic medicine was already extensively developed by the time of Gautama Buddha, and the Buddha supported both the study and the practice of medicine. Since the days of Charaka and Sushruta, Ayurvedic students started dissecting human corpses, practicing the arts of surgery on dummies, and learning other practical arts such as cookery (since diet was an essential aspect of treatment), the collection and preparation of herbs, horticulture, and the purification and preparation of mineral medicines. Each student usually specialized in one of Ayurveda's eight "limbs": Internal Medicine, surgery, eye-ear-nose, gynecology-obstetrics-pediatrics, psychology, toxicology, rejuvenation, and virilization. At the end of the period of study, the disciple was thoroughly tested, and after graduation was given a license to practice by the king.

After Ashoka, the emperor of most of North India about three centuries before the birth of Christ, embraced Buddhism, he furnished extensive support to medicine and built charitable hospitals including specialized surgical, obstetric and mental facilities throughout his realm for both humans and animals, and his emissaries spread Buddhism and Indian sciences in far-off lands including Central Asia and Sri Lanka. During the later Indian empires of the Guptas and the Mauryas, the government expanded this active support for medicine by planting gardens of medicinal herbs, establishing hospitals and maternity homes, posting physicians in villages, and punishing quacks who tried to practice medicine without proper learning and imperial license.

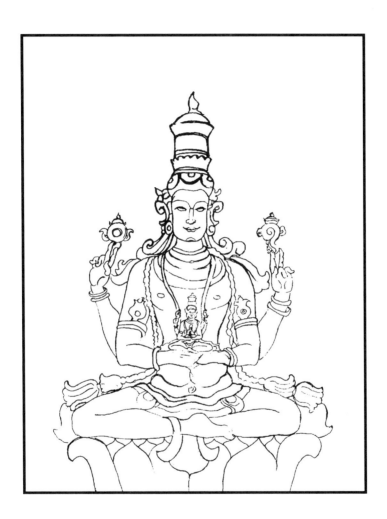

8. Dhanvantari

Dhanvantari is described in many texts as the patron god of physicians and surgeons, who appeared during the primordial churning of the ocean carrying divine nectar. He is also considered to be a minor incarnation of Vishnu (embodiment of compassion). The *Bhava Prakasha* (a medical text) describes him as the physician of the gods: according to the text, he was directed by Indra, the king of the gods, to visit mankind as a physician and eliminate suffering.

During this era Ayurveda was taught in large Buddhist universities like the one at Nalanda, established during the fourth century A.D. and which flourished for about eight hundred years. Students came from all over the world to study at these universities. More texts appeared, including Vagbhata's *Ashtanga Sangraha* (*Collected Teachings of the Eight Limbs*) and *Ashtanga Hrdaya* (*Heart of the Eight Limbs*). These are condensations of Charaka and Sushruta's teachings, and Madhava's *Madhava Nidana* (*Text on Diagnosis*). Ayurveda was not limited to humans; texts on the treatment of trees, horses and elephants still exist, and may have existed for such varied animals as cows, goats, sheep, donkeys, camels and hawks.

The Golden Age of Indian culture ended when Muslim invaders inundated Northern India after the tenth century. They slaughtered the Buddhist monks as infidels, destroyed the universities and burned the libraries. Those who could escape fled to Nepal and Tibet, and hence some Ayurvedic texts whose originals were lost at that time survive solely in the Tibetan translation. Though the Muslim conquerors imported their own system of medicine into India, fortunately Ayurveda did survive as did the Hindu culture. In the thirteenth or fourteenth century a treatise on Ayurvedic pharmacology, the *Sharngadhara Samhita*, appeared, and during the sixteenth century all Indian medical knowledge was collected and compiled by the order of the Mughal Emperor Akbar.

The conquests of the Europeans, however, were nearly fatal to Ayurveda, especially after 1835 when the British decided neither to recognize nor support Indian sciences in their Indian dominions. While the Germans, and later other Westerners developed plastic surgery from Sushruta's operation for repair of damaged noses and ears, it took the upsurge of Indian Nationalism at the beginning of this century to reawaken interest in the native Indian arts and sciences in India itself. Ayurveda began its renaissance then, and today it is one of the six medical systems in India which is officially recognized by India's government, the others being Allopathy, Unani, Siddha, Homeopathy and Naturopathy.

2
The Sankhya Philosophy

The evolution of the universe as detailed in the Sankhya system, one of the six systems of philosophy in India, forms the foundation for most Ayurvedic theories. Yoga uses the same approach with only minor alterations. In the Sankhya philosophy, everything evolves from an Absolute Reality (purusha) which is consciousness without any characteristic whatsoever, beyond time, space, and causation, a single point which encompasses everything and which cannot be perceived by mind or accurately described in human language. All potentialities exist within Absolute Reality in an unmanifested state. From this Absolute Reality evolves Relative Reality, a sublime creative force called Nature (prakriti). The sole difference between Nature and Absolute Reality is that the Absolute knows itself to be identical to Nature, whereas Nature believes itself to be different from the Absolute. This passive awareness of difference then evolves into a undifferentiated Intelligence (mahat), a faculty through which this difference is actively perceived. Intelligence is thus Nature's unlimited self-awareness. This undifferentiated Intelligence then individuates into discrete bundles of limited self-awareness called Ego (ahamkara). Each of these is self-aware, but aware only of that limited parcel of being with which it identifies.

Nature, as manifested through individual bundles of Ego, has Three Attributes (gunas): Sattva (equilibrium), Rajas (activity) and Tamas (inertia). Rajas is movement, Tamas matter, and Sattva that subjectivity which perceives matter. Sattva evolves into the thinking mind, the five senses of perception and the five senses of action (communication, manipulation, locomotion, procreation and excretion, represented in the human body by voice, hands, feet, genitals and anus respectively). Tamas evolves into the objects of the cognitive senses—sound, touch, form, taste and odor—which in turn produce the Five Great Elements (pancha mahabhutas) which make up the physical universe: Ether, Air, Fire, Water and Earth. Rajas is the force which brings the senses and their objects together. I go to sleep as "I" at night and wake up as "I" the next morning because Ahamkara identifies "I" with a particular body, a certain set of habits and preferences, and specific desires and disgusts. Sattva, Rajas and Tamas are the three powers through which Ahamkara creates self-image (see illustration 9).

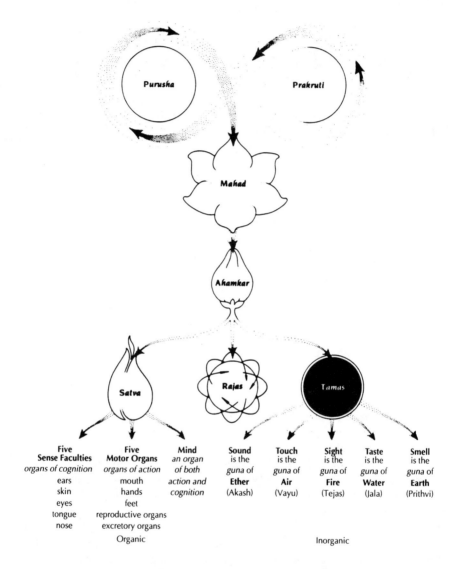

Five Sense Faculties	Five Motor Organs	Mind	Sound	Touch	Sight	Taste	Smell
organs of cognition	*organs of action*	*an organ*	is the	is the	is the	is the	is the
		of both	*guna* of	*guna* of	*guna* of	*guna* of	*guna* of
ears	mouth	*action and*	**Ether**	**Air**	**Fire**	**Water**	**Earth**
skin	hands	*cognition*	(Akash)	(Vayu)	(Tejas)	(Jala)	(Prithvi)
eyes	feet						
tongue	reproductive organs						
nose	excretory organs						
	Organic				Inorganic		

9. Samkhya Philosophy of Creation

Purusha is unmanifested, formless, passive, beyond attributes, beyond cause and effect, space and time. Purusha is Pure Existence. **Prakruti** is the creative force of action, the source of form, manifestation, attributes and nature. **Mahad** is the Cosmic Intelligence or Buddhi. **Ahamkar** is ego, the sense of "I Am." **Satva** is stability, pure aspect, awakening, essence and light. **Rajas** is dynamic movement. **Tamas** is static; it is potential energy, inertia, darkness, ignorance and matter.

The Five Great Elements are really states of matter: Earth is the solid state, Water the liquid state, Air the gaseous state, Fire the power to change the state of any substance, and Ether the field which is both the source of all matter and the space in which it exists. Ether is the most rarefied stage of matter and Earth the solidest. Every substance in our world is made up of these Five Elements and can be classified according to which Element is predominant. Things which are solid under normal conditions are composed primarily of the Earth Element, substances which are normally gases are mainly composed of Air, and anything which is usually liquid is mainly made of Water. Reactive or unstable substances are usually Fiery in nature, and Ether predominance in a substance is shown by its rarefaction or lack of density.

Our physical bodies are also made up of these Five Great Elements; in fact, the Law of Microcosm and Macrocosm (according to the *Charaka Samhita*) states that everything that exists in the vast external universe, the macrocosm, also appears in the internal cosmos of the human body, the microcosm, in altered form. The universe is thus continually influencing us, and likewise we influence it. Prana, Subtle Fire (tejas) and Essence (ojas) are the quintessential expressions of the Five Elements as applied to embodied life. Furthermore, Prana, Subtle Fire and Essence individually express the intrinsic attributes of Air, Fire and Water Elements, respectively, in their greatest degree. Prana is the life force, the power which holds body, mind and spirit together and compels them to function together. Prana is not air, though oxygen is one of its vehicles. Subtle Fire causes the transformations necessary to allow influences to pass from one plane of existence to another, and Essence is the subtle glue which cements body, mind and spirit together, integrating them into a functioning individual.

3
The Three Doshas

*P*rana, Subtle Fire and Essence are too subtle to satisfy all of a living body's energy requirements and so they metamorphose into doshas, a dosha being a fault or error, a thing which can go wrong. The Three Doshas inside a living body—Vata, Pitta and Kapha—are grosser forms of Prana, Subtle Fire and Essence respectively. They, too, are condensed from the Five Great Elements: Vata arises from Air and Ether, Pitta from Fire and Water, and Kapha from Water and Earth. Therefore each Dosha is comprised of two Elements; one functions as its active component while the other acts as the passive medium through which the active element is expressed. Thus Vata, Pitta and Kapha are most representative of Air, Fire and Water, respectively.

All movements of any kind in the physical body of every living being in our world are governed by Vata. All transformations of every kind, and particularly those involving digestion of food and information, are governed by Pitta. Stability, including such functions as lubrication of joints and organs, is governed by Kapha. Though direct perception of these Doshas, which do not exist on the physical plane is not possible, it is possible to discern their presence and influence by examining their effects on the organism. Bile, phlegm and other bodily secretions are vehicles for the Three Doshas, substances through which they display their qualities and perform their actions. All Five Elements are essential to life, and their harmony, which arises when Vata, Pitta and Kapha are balanced, determines an individual's condition of health or disease. A healthy organism produces just enough of the Three Doshas to meet physical needs, while an unhealthy body overproduces or underproduces the Doshas at the expense of the body's vitality, adaptability and immunity.

Whether a substance increases or decreases a Dosha depends upon the Law of Like and Unlike, according to the *Charaka Samhita*. "Like increases like" means that when you eat, drink, inhale or otherwise imbibe a substance, the qualities of that substance increase those parts of your system which possess similar qualities. Substances which are mainly composed of Earth and Water will increase the body's proportion of Earth and Water and will therefore increase Kapha, constituted of Earth and Water. For example, ice cream being mainly composed of Earth and Water and being cold, heavy, wet, sticky and dense increases body constituents with like qualities, e.g. mucus. Ten pairs of qualities are commonly recognized in Ayurvedic analyses of substances:

> heavy and light
> cold and hot
> wet and dry
> dull and acute
> stable and mobile
> soft and hard
> clear and sticky
> smooth and rough
> subtle and gross
> solid and liquid

What is unlike a thing tends to reduce it; black pepper, for example, is hot, light, and dry; is not sticky or dense, and thus tends to decrease the body's mucus. Whether ice cream will be better for you than black pepper or not depends upon what your system requires to remain in balance at any particular moment. A substance can exert three possible effects on an organism: it can act as food and nourish it, act as medicine and harmonize it, or act as poison and derange it.

The Three Doshas, like the Elements from which they arise, increase and decrease in the body according to the qualities present in the body; qualities which we absorb from our food, drink and our environment, and derive through our intrinsic chemistry. Even our thoughts and emotions have qualities that affect the body's Doshas. Each of these Doshas has its own set of qualities:

> **Vata** is dry, cold, light, unstable, clear, rough, and subtle;
> **Pitta** is slightly oily, hot, intense, light, fluid, malodorous (a raw-meat-like smell), and mobile;
> **Kapha** is oily, cold, heavy, stable, viscid, smooth, and soft.

Whatever goes into the system influences the system with its characteristics. The most important of all inputs is food which affects the system thrice: before digestion when it is tasted by the tongue, during digestion while it moves through the gut, and after digestion when it passes into the tissues. These effects are called taste, potency and post-digestive effect respectively.

Six tastes are described in Ayurveda: sweet, sour, salty, pungent, bitter and astringent (see illustration 10). Sweet, sour and salty tend to increase Kapha and decrease Vata; pungent, bitter and astringent exert precisely the opposite action, increasing Vata and decreasing Kapha. Sweet, bitter and astringent relieve Pitta, while sour, salty and pungent increase it. These tastes are derived from the Five Elements; each a composite of two elements in the same manner as the Doshas. Sweet is composed of earth and water; licorice root is a good example of a substance that is primarily

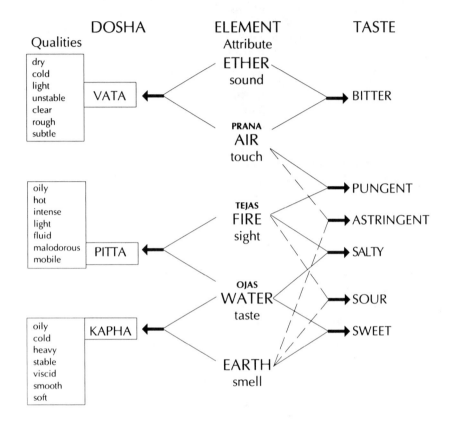

10. Primal Elements
Attributes and Relationships to DOSHAS and TASTES

sweet in taste. The sour taste, as of hibiscus, is made up of earth and fire. Water and fire combine to form the salty taste; which appears mainly in salt and seaweeds. Pungent substances like chilies and cloves are mainly composed of air and fire. Gentian and barberry are examples of plants which are predominantly bitter in taste with air and ether as the main elements. Witch hazel and unripe persimmons are mainly astringent; in these air and earth dominate.

Although the pairs of strong potencies include heavy/light and wet/dry, the most important duality is that of hot and cold. Hot food enhances the fire available to the body, while cold food reduces it. Generally sour, salty and pungent substances are hot while sweet, bitter and astringent substances are cold.

There are three types of post-digestive effects derived from the natural qualities of the food and the strength of the digestive process: sweet tends to expand the tissues, enhances Kapha, and builds up the body; sour increases Pitta and may burn away the tissues; and pungent augments Vata and dries out the tissues. In general, sweet and salty substances lead to a sweet post-digestive effect, while sour substances lead to a sour one, and bitter, pungent and astringent substances result in a pungent post-digestive effect (see illustration 11).

Certain foods, medicines, and poisons possess specialized attributes or powers (prabhava). When a substance possessing a special power is consumed, it may produce unusual effects in the body and mind, effects which cannot be predicted by the classificatory knowledge of taste, potency or post-digestive effect.

Charaka, in summarizing the ideal attributes of a medicinal substance, says: "A medicine is one which enters the body, balances the Doshas, does not disturb the healthy tissue, does not adhere to them and gets eliminated through the urine, sweat and feces. It cures the disease, gives longevity to the bodily cells and has no side effects."

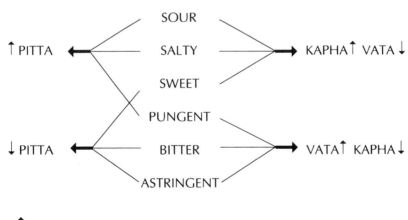

↑ this dosha is enhanced
↓ this dosha is decreased

11. Correlation of Doshas with Tastes

4

The Doshas in the Body

The Three Doshas pervade the entire body but concentrate only in those tissues in which they are particularly required. Thus Vata accumulates below the navel to help counteract the force of gravity by pumping blood, lymph and wastes from the lower parts of the body back into the torso; whereas Kapha accumulates above the diaphragm to keep Vata from moving upward too strongly, and to ensure lubrication for those organs which require it most (the heart, lungs and alimentary canal); and Pitta, the mediator and fulcrum between Vata and Kapha, occupies the region between the diaphragm and the navel, near the body's center of gravity.

Certain body organs generally store higher concentrations of each of the Doshas:

VATA—brain and nervous system, heart, large intestine, bones, lungs, bladder, pelvis, thighs, ears and skin.

PITTA—brain, liver, spleen, gallbladder, small intestine, endocrine glands, skin, eyes, blood and sweat.

KAPHA—brain, joints, mouth, head and neck, stomach, lymph, chest (especially lungs, heart and esophagus), kidneys and fat.

Vata, Pitta and Kapha each has five particularized aspects. The five Kaphas manifest in specialized body lubricants such as stomach mucus, pleural and pericardial fluid, saliva, synovial fluid, and cerebrospinal fluid. The five Pittas appear in transformative substances including digestive juices, hemoglobin, melanin, rhodopsin, and various neurotransmitters. The five Vatas divide the body into spheres of influence as follows:

The field of activity of Forward-Moving (prana) Vata extends from the diaphragm to the throat; it is in charge of taking in of things like food, water and air, into the system. All five Vatas are derived from Prana, but since this Vata is particularly involved with the intake of the life force itself, it has been ascribed this name.

The field of Upward-Moving (udana) Vata extends from the throat to the top of the head, and it controls self-expression: speech, endeavor, enthusiasm, memory, vitality, complexion (one of the body's means of expressing its innate state) and the like.

The Downward-Moving (apana) Vata, operates from the navel to the anus. It expels things from the body: urine, feces, gas, semen, menstrual blood, and the fetus.

The Pervasive (vyana) Vata pervades the entire body from its seat in the heart, distributing nourishment by causing blood and other fluids to circulate and producing locomotion, extension and contraction, perspiration, and other similar actions.

The field of Equalizing (samana) Vata extends from the diaphragm to the navel. It directs the processes of digestion and assimilation, and helps keep Forward-Moving and Downward-Moving Vatas balanced.

Vata, Pitta and Kapha act through the body's tissues and waste products. Actually it is the Doshas which really make the body function, since the tissues are arranged and nourished and the wastes sequestered and excreted by the Doshas. A human being is a factory in which raw materials are operated upon by the Doshas to produce products and by-products. While the building, the machines and the raw materials are all essential ingredients for production of goods; without the workers (the Doshas) there is no production! The products of digestion are the seven tissues which anchor mind and spirit firmly to the physical body. They are Sap (rasa), Blood (rakta), Flesh (mamsa), Fat (medas), Bone (asthi), Marrow (majja) and Reproductive Tissue (shukra) (see illustration 12).

Sap (rasa), the foundation of the body, is the first "juice" absorbed from the digested food; it includes but is not limited to chyle. Sushruta emphasized Sap's importance thus: "Knowing that humans are the product of Rasa, one must be specially careful about the preservation of Rasa." Each tissue acts as the raw material for the next; that is, Blood is formed from Sap, Flesh from Blood, Fat from Flesh, and so on. At each stage of transformation the next tissue in the sequence is produced along with a waste and a secondary tissue.

Reproductive Tissue includes all the body's reproductive fluids, male and female; it produces no waste, and its secondary tissue is the fetus it creates. The action of a very subtle form of Fire on Reproductive Tissue generates Essence (ojas), the glandular secretion which cements body, mind and spirit together. Although semen is produced in the testicles, the energy which that semen carries comes from Bone and Marrow. Since Reproductive Tissue is the raw material from which Essence is produced, excessive loss of Reproductive Tissue depletes Essence, weakening immunity and digestive capacity. When Essence is firm the mind is firm; excessive sex robs the mind of its firmness because Essence and Reproductive Tissue are continually lost. It takes time for ingested food to proceed through the tissues to nourish Reproductive Tissue, though milk, honey, onions and alchemically prepared mercury are some of the substances reported to replenish the body's Reproductive Tissue almost instantly.

Essence is both the cause and the effect of good digestion, and its conservation is essential to good health because it controls the immune system and generates the body's aura, the halo of lustre which is the essence of one's being. Lustre which is "expansive, glossy and broad" is auspicious, while a "dry, soiled or contracted" lustre betokens inauspiciousness and disease.

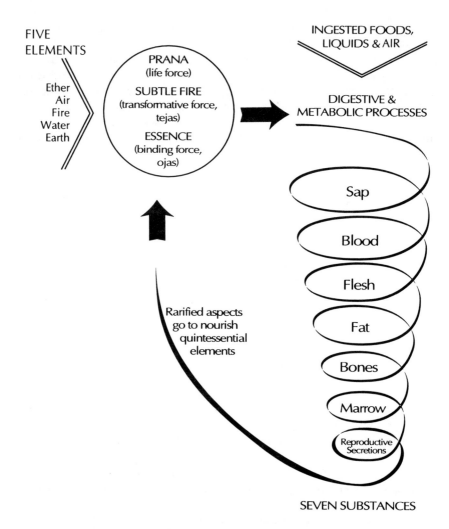

12. The Seven Substances

The Five Elements are expressed in embodied life as Prana, Subtle Fire (tejas) and Essence (ojas) which act upon the digestive and metabolic processes to produce seven substances. In progressive order the substances appear as: Sap, Blood, Flesh, Fat, Bones, Marrow, and Reproductive Secretions. Their prime purpose is to build up and sustain the body, while rarefied aspects serve reciprocally to nourish the Prana, Subtle Fire and Essence.

5
Channels of Flow

When balanced the Doshas support the body by irrigating the tissues with Sap (rasa) as water irrigates a field. Like crops in a field the tissues require channels through which the nutrient juices can flow to reach them. The body possesses many Channels (srotamsi), large and small, through which nutrients and wastes move. Many of these channels, such as the digestive tract, look like pipes even to the naked eye, while others are less tube-like. The digestive tract is the most important of all the bodily channels, since it takes in the Elements necessary to replenish body tissues and maintain the system's continuity.

Though innumerable, fourteen of these channels are primary. Three of them deal with nutrition from outside: the Prana Channel, composed of the respiratory system and the heart; the Water Channel, which extends from the palate to the pancreas; and the Food Channel, extending from the esophagus to the large intestine. Seven channels deal with tissue nutrition: the Sap Channel consists of the heart and its great vessels, the Blood Channel is based in the liver and spleen, the Flesh Channel consists of the muscles and skin, the Fat Channel includes the kidneys and omentum, the Bone Channel consists of the fat and the hips, the Marrow Channel consists of the bones, the joints and everything which is encased within bone, and the Reproductive Tissue Channel consists of the testes and penis in the male and their corresponding structures (the ovaries, vagina and clitoris) in the female. Three more channels deal with the elimination of wastes: the Urine Channel consists of the bladder and kidneys, the Feces Channel of the colon and rectum, and the Sweat Channel of the fat and hair follicles.

The fourteenth channel, the Channel of Mind, pervades the entire body; the body is in a sense the mind's special channel. There is nowhere in the body mind cannot and does not go. Two more channels are peculiar to the female: the Milk Channel and the Menstrual Channel, both of which are secondary to the Sap Channel. The Milk Channel includes the breasts and nipples, and the Menstrual Channel the uterus, cervix and vagina. When all flows are regular in the various channels the organism is healthy and therefore happy, just as when a field is well-watered its crops grow well. Should the circulation in any channel become obstructed, nutrients and/or wastes will accumulate and cause the bodily equivalent of a flooded field, yielding imbalance and disease. There are four possible disturbances to flow in a channel: increase or decrease in flow, a "knotted" condition (obstruction), and deviation of its flow into abnormal spaces. Any disturbance to a channel's flow will disturb Vata.

One important cause of such disturbances is due to the restraining of the thirteen urges, namely the urges to: expel urine, feces, and flatus; vomit, sneeze, belch, and yawn; eat when hungry, drink when thirsty, cry when sad, sleep when sleepy, pant after exertion, and ejaculate semen when irresistibly aroused. Restraint of these urges causes Vata to move in an abnormal direction in these channels, vitiating first the channel involved and then the entire system. Other urges even though not physical reflexes can still disturb Vata. These include especially the negative mental urges like greed, sorrow, fear, anger, envy, pride, shame, disgust, and the like, and ought always to be restrained, though not suppressed.

6
Subtle Anatomy

*T*he human body is composed of a number of intricately interwoven layers, like an onion, among which are the changeable body of fluids, including the tissues and wastes; the relatively less changeable body of muscles, bones, and nerves; the subtle body, which is the field of mind; and the causal body. Though we cannot dissect these "bodies" apart from one another, we call them "bodies" because in certain ways they behave as if they were separate structures within the unified organism. These layers or Sheaths (kosas) are generated as consciousness descends into denser and denser matter, with the subtler Sheaths acting as patterns for the grosser ones. It is as if each level of organization tries to reproduce the previous level, but cannot do so precisely because of the increased density of the matter it must work with.

The physical body is the Sheath of Food; it is composed of and nourished by the juices extracted from our food. The Sheath of Prana, the vital body, connects the Sheaths of Food and Mind and permits them to operate together. It is composed of and nourished by Prana alone. Prana is "energy," but it is also a form of matter when viewed in the context of consciousness. The organism's Prana is replenished in two ways: "instantly" in which the lungs during breathing absorb the Prana found in the air, and "delayed," in which the large intestine absorbs the Prana found in well-digested food. The Sheath of Mind is the astral body, which is composed of and nourished by words, images and emotions, all of which are made out of "mind-stuff," a very subtle form of matter.

The role of the Sheath of Food, in which Tamas predominates, is the stabilization of consciousness, while the Sheath of Prana, in which Rajas predominates, is meant to activate it. The job of the Sheath of Mind is to mediate between the other Sheaths to ensure that the Prana and the physical body remain in balance with the mind. Since an excess of either Rajas (overactivity) or Tamas (inertia) will disturb its balance, Rajas and Tamas are called the mind's Doshas, and when either appears in excess the mind becomes deranged. When the Three Doshas of the body become imbalanced they can also imbalance the mind; the mental and physical Doshas interact with and affect one another continuously by way of Prana, the force which binds them together. Mind, Prana and body are concurrently and inherently joined together as long as life continues in a body.

In the physical body energy and fluids move through visible channels (like the nerves and blood vessels), while in the vital body Prana moves through the subtle conduits and plexuses called Nadis and Chakras, respectively. The vital or Pranic body exerts its effects by stimulating the physical channels which flow in synchrony with its Nadis. The body's most important Nadi, which is also the least used by the average individual, is called the Central Conduit (sushumna). The Chakras are arranged like flowers in a garland along the thread of the Central Conduit, which flows within the central sulcus of the spinal cord—or it would do so if it existed on the physical plane! More precisely the Central Conduit flows through the same space which on the physical level is taken up by the central sulcus of the spinal cord. Since these two structures exist on different levels of being they can occupy the same space simultaneously, an impulse in one often engendering an impulse in the other by resonance.

The body's next two most important Nadis (ida and pingala) flow in conjunction with the two nostrils. Most of the time we breathe only through one nostril, shifting unconsciously from right to left and back every two to three hours. The left nostril (or rather its Nadi, the pingala) cools and calms the organism, while the right (ida) heats and excites it. Heat expands, and cold contracts; in the body of a living being heat generally dilates the channels and cold constricts them. These two Nadis govern and maintain the rhythmic contraction and expansion of the body and its physiology, a heat-cold duality which fuels the circulation of Vata in the body very much as the dance of hot and cold air masses fuels the circulation of atmospheric air. Excess or lack of heat in the body obstructs Vata's movement and predisposes to disease. Physicians who use the esoteric form of diagnosis, called "svarodaya" in Sanskrit, detect the subtle differences in the direction and rate of flow of the breath in their own nostrils to indicate the condition of the flow of Prana in their patient's Nadis.

While most of the Nadis work in consonance with body structures, Central Conduit and its Chakras reside in a plane of existence so subtle that the average human being never suspects their presence. The Chakras, which exist in the Central Conduit, function only when Prana flows through that Nadi, and unless energy is actually flowing through a Chakra it cannot really be even said to exist, remaining instead in an inactive, potential form.

Many sensitive people report that they can see "energy vortices", "spinning patterns" and other concentrations of power within the living human body. While it is true that such flows often exist near in space to the regions were the Chakras are said to be located, all such flows appear in the layers of the organism that are superficial to the Chakras. Only the most spiritually advanced of beings can directly perceive the Chakras.

The body possesses many potential Chakras in whose region varying amounts of energy may concentrate. Six major Chakras are generally agreed upon, however: at the perineum; sex center; solar plexus; heart; throat; and between the eyebrows. The energy center on top of the head, known as the "Thousand-Petalled Lotus" (sahasrara) is not a Chakra; it marks the boundary between the region of the microcosm in which the Prana is restricted to moving within the Nadis, and the region of the macrocosm, where the Prana has "thousands" of paths in which to move. Each of the five principal lower Chakras connects the organism to a specific Element. Speech, a function of the Ether Element (which has sound as its special quality), manifests at the throat. The Air Element, which moves incessantly, is concentrated in the chest, the home of the ever-mobile heart and lungs. The digestive organs, liver and spleen, all "hot" organs, cluster around the area near the solar plexus generated by the Fire Element. The Water Element, without which no life exists, is responsible for the genitals. The Earth Element, the foundation of physical existence, is located at the perineum, the foundation of the torso. This lowest Chakra, the home of Mother Earth, is the lower pole of an axis whose upper pole, the "Sky-Father," lies within the brain, just as Earth and Sky are the two poles of the macrocosm (see illustration 13).

The Nadis direct the activity of the physical channels through which energy flows, including the nerves, bones, joints, muscles, ligaments and glands, which then move the body's juices around. This system like any system is weakest at those points where things join together. A Marma is a point on the human body beneath which vital channels intersect. Some of these intersections are physically identifiable while others are subtle structures. Some Marma points are identical with acupuncture points and others are nearly identical. Since Vedic times warriors in India targeted Marmas on the bodies of their enemies to inflict maximal damage and surgeons used their knowledge of Marmas to treat such injuries. The *Sushruta Samhita*, Ayurveda's surgical text, classifies 107 Marmas on the basis of the structure (muscles, blood vessels, ligaments, nerves, bones, joints), on the regional location, the dimension, and the consequences of injury (swift death, death after some delay, death as soon as any foreign body is extracted from the wound, disability, or simply intense pain) (see illustration 14).

In the southern state of Kerala the practitioners of the martial art known as kalarippayattu (see illustration 19 in Part 3), which like Hatha Yoga involves a set of preliminary physical exercises that lead both to physical and mental control, recognize 160 to 220 Marmas in martial practice, and use the 107 Marmas of Sushruta in therapy. According to kalarippayattu, injury to a Marma blocks or cuts the associated Nadi at that point, interrupting both the flow of Prana—the life force, and the flow of Vata—Prana's waste product and servant, in that area. For serious damage to occur a blow must penetrate an inch or more into the tissues

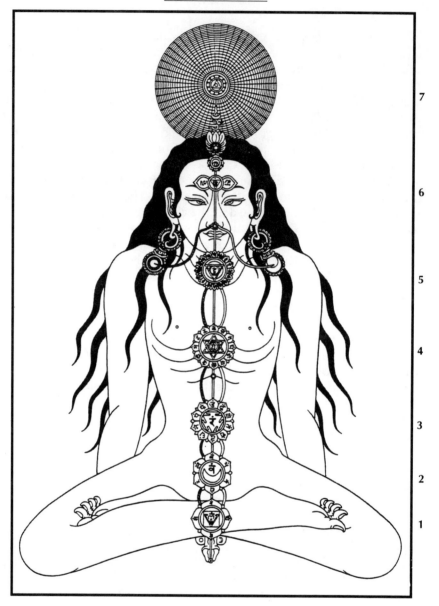

13. The Nadis and Chakras

Nadis
Figure's left side: Ida (Pingala)
Center: Sushumna-Central Conduit
Figure's right side: Pingala (Ida)

Chakras (in ascending order)
1. Muladhara-Earth 2. Svadhishthana-Water
3. Manipura-Fire 4. Anahata-Air
5. Vishuddha-Ether 6. Ajna-Duality
7. Sahasrara (Thousand-petalled Lotus)

This drawing shows the approximate location of the three main Nadis and the six major Chakras within the physical body. The Central Conduit (sushumna) lies in between the two Nadis (ida and pingala) linked with the nostrils. The Chakras are situated within the Central Conduit; they are traditionally represented by elements and symbols as seen in this depiction.

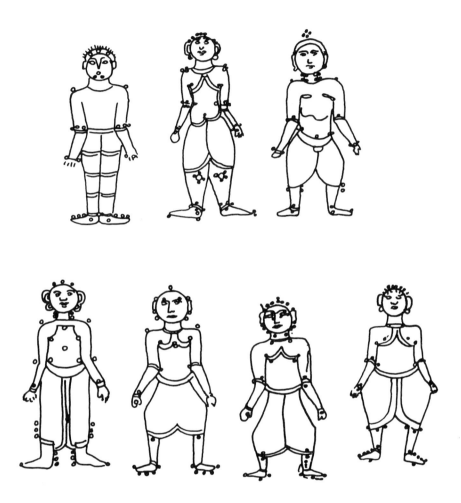

14. Ancient Marma Figures

Seven figures showing the various points locations (called nilas in Sinhalese or marmas in Sanskrit) amenable for needling and cauterization therapy according to traditional Sinhala medicine of Sri Lanka.

beneath the spot; a mere slap will not be so harmful. An immediate anti-dote for such an injury is a firm stroke or slap to the similar Marma on the opposite side of the body which gets the Prana moving again. Such a counter-application must be given within a specified time in order to work, and must then be followed by treatment for the imbalance of the Doshas caused by the injury.

Like a Chakra, a Marma is not really a "structure" in that it does not exist at all times. Marmas exists only insofar as there is Prana in the body—that is, a dead body has no Marma within it—and any Marma is only activated fully when Prana is actually moving in it; the death or damage predicted for injury to a Marma occurs only when such a Marma is active. Prana's movement through and concentration in the body's Marmas is controlled by the lunar day. In this the doctrine of Marma is strikingly similar to that of Indian sexology, which details the specific ar-eas of a woman's body which are awake to erotic excitement on particu-lar lunar days because of the movement of Prana therein. Vata's gati (cog-nate with the English word "gait") is defined as both its way of moving through the body and the direction taken by this movement. Diagnosis is a report on the path taken by the system's Vata and other Doshas, and re-turn of Vata's gait to normal is an essential part of any therapy.

7
Constitution

*E*veryone has a typical rhythm, an innate gait, determined by our genes and chromosomes. A human's gait, like an animal's, reflects the body's internal energy equation. All of us tend to favor particular energy pathways, organs, glands, nerves, limbs, thoughts and images. The sum total of this preference produces our own individual gaits. Ayurveda calls a person's characteristic physical and mental constitution, prakriti, to be distinguished from vikriti—the condition or current state of a person's health which differs from moment to moment. The sages used the word prakriti advisedly since it also means the manifested universe as a whole, and a person's constitution is a representation of that person's intimate universe.

Personal constitution, which is fixed at the moment of conception, is determined by conditions prevailing in the bodies and minds of the child's parents at that time. If, for example, during sexual intercourse the force of Kapha was increased in the father and Vata predominated in the mother, the child will always be, all through its life, constitutionally prone to over-activity of both Kapha and Vata. Pitta will still be present, as it is in all living beings, but its role will be less prominent. Severe disease may make the underlying constitution irrelevant to diagnosis, but that pattern is etched permanently into the genetic material. The diet and activity of the mother during pregnancy, conditions in the womb during pregnancy, and events during delivery may also influence the child's subsequent health and happiness, but these are all secondary to constitution.

There are eight principal constitution types:

(1) Balanced: in which all three Doshas tend to remain in equilibrium.
(2) Vata: in which Vata is significantly stronger than both Pitta and Kapha.
(3) Pitta: in which Pitta is significantly stronger than both Vata and Kapha.
(4) Kapha: in which Kapha is significantly stronger than both Pitta and Vata.
(5) Vata-Pitta or Pitta-Vata: in which these two Doshas are both significantly stronger than Kapha, though one of them

may be slightly stronger relative to the other.

(6) Pitta-Kapha or Kapha-Pitta: in which these two Doshas are both significantly stronger than Vata, though one of them may be somewhat stronger relative to the other.

(7) Vata-Kapha or Kapha-Vata: in which these two Doshas are both significantly stronger than Pitta, and one of them may be slightly stronger relative to the other.

(8) Imbalanced: in which the three Doshas tend to go out of equilibrium altogether.

Most people have double predominance, though considering the possible permutations of the degree of predominance of these Doshas the number of constitutional types becomes infinite. People are classified by constitution to help them select appropriate habits and lifestyles to enhance health maintenance. The accompanying chart (illustration 15) details the constitutional attributes of the three main Doshas.

CHARACTERISTIC	VATA	PITTA	KAPHA
Body Frame	narrow, disproportionate	medium, usually proportionate	broad, well proportioned
Weight	easy to lose, hard to gain	easy to lose, easy to gain	hard to lose, easy to gain
Skin	dark or tans easily, often cool to the touch	light, sunburns easily, often warm to the touch	medium shade, tans easily, often cool to the touch
Sweat	scanty, even in heat	profuse in heat	moderate, consistent
Hair	dry, coarse, curly, often dark	fine, light in color, often straight, may be oily, grays or balds early	oily, lustrous, thick, usually brown
Eye color	often gray, or violet	often hazel, green, or blue	brown, occasionally blue
Appetite	variable	intense	regular
Evacuation	erratic, often constipated	usually regular, sometimes loose	regular, slow
Climate	prefers warm	prefers cool	enjoys changes of season
Stamina	poor, tends to over-exert	medium, over-exerts when competing	good, but tends to under-exert
Sex drive	variable	often intense	steady
Fertility	often poor	medium	usually good
Sleep	variable, often poor; deep when fatigued	sleeps and rises easily	sleeps easily, rises with reluctance
Speech	talkative, may ramble	speaks with a purpose	slow, cautious
Emotion	fear often prevalent	tends to anger easily	likes to avoid confrontation
Thinking	usually verbal imagery	much visual imagery	images arise mainly from feelings and emotions
Memory	learns and forgets quickly	learns quickly, forgets slowly	learns and forgets slowly

15. Doshas and Constitution

8
Disease Causation

According to Ayurveda there are basically three types of diseases: endogenous (breakdowns from within), exogenous (attacks from without), and mental; any of which can subsequently lead to others. The tissues and wastes are the "things" in the body which are vitiated by the Doshas, the vitiation spreading from one tissue or waste to other tissues. Disturbed channels spread their corruption only to other body channels and polluted tissues to other tissues alone, "whereas Vata, Pitta and Kapha when vitiated pollute the entire organism, being, as they are, of a vitiating nature."

Time, like personal constitution, is one of the more significant factors implicated in the generation of disease. Diseases are said to arise at the "junctions" of the seasons. This applies literally to the junctions of winter with spring (Kapha aggravation), spring with summer (Pitta inflammation) and summer with fall (Vata disturbance). This is because the body must adapt to changing external conditions, but becomes imbalanced if the adaptation is less than perfect. It also applies to other "seasons" of one's life: the day, age, and digestion. After eating and before digestion actually begins, Kapha predominates; Pitta dominates during digestion; and during assimilation Vata predominates. Youth (birth to the end of bone growth) is the Kapha time of life; adulthood (end of youth to menopause or the male equivalent) is the Pitta period; and during the senior years Vata rules. Kapha predominates for roughly the first third of the day (i.e. sunrise to midmorning) and the first third of the night (sunset to late evening), Pitta for the middle thirds of the day and the night, and Vata for the last thirds of day and night (i.e. the periods just before sunrise and sunset) (see illustration 16).

No single factor is wholly responsible for either health or disease; they are the result of the concerted action of many causes. Since however all diseases to some degree disturb a proper functioning of the Three Doshas, diseases are usually classified according to the underlying causative Dosha. Most causes of disease are individual and preventable, but most of us fail to prevent the diseases by acting contrary to what we know is in our own self-interest mainly, due to a weakness of the mental will. Every one of us must "digest" all the sense perceptions which inundate us.

DOSHA	JUNCTION OF SEASON	DIGESTION	AGE	DAY CYCLE
Kapha	Winter-Spring	before	youth	after sunrise & sunset
Pitta	Spring-Summer	during	adulthood	noon & midnight
Vata	Summer-Fall	after	old age	before sunrise & sunset

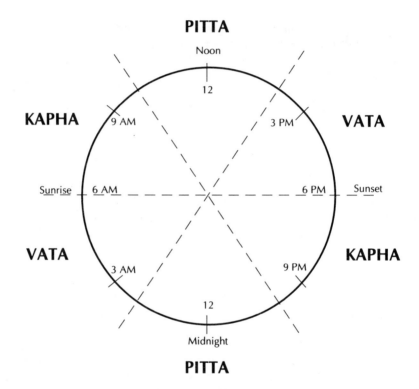

16. Doshas and Time Factors

This table indicates the times when each dosha is naturally increased as a result of time changes. It is only an approximation, because the relative length of Kapha, Pitta, and Vata periods tend to vary with the length of the day. Also how these time periods will be experienced will vary from individual to individual.

When the temptation to enjoy a thing or the desire to avoid another, overwhelms our innate common sense and leads us to perform actions resulting in an imbalance of the Doshas, it should be clear to us that our mental "digestion" (the ability to know what is appropriate and what is inappropriate for health) has become disturbed. This violation of good sense or perversity of mind, which arises from attempts to rearrange the world to suit oneself while ignoring the inherent rhythm of the universe, is known as prajnaparadha, meaning literally, "a transgression against wisdom." Such sins of omission or commission are the ultimate causes of all pathological conditions, and can affect any activity of speech, mind or body, directly or indirectly. Such transgressions usually involve either improper use of the sense organs or inattention to the changes in diet and lifestyle necessitated by daily, seasonal or other time cycles.

All diseases are due either to under-nourishment (drying out the body) or over-nourishment (making it too wet). Substances and activities which cause the "wetness" of the system to increase weaken the digestive fire in the same way that wetness weakens an external fire. Most diseases in affluent societies are due to excess of wetness because most affluent people over-consume everything. The poor, and those people who deliberately under-consume (through prolonged fasting, anorexia, bulimia and the like), develop diseases of under-nourishment. Because dryness is a characteristic of Vata, the drying out of the body by under-nourishment usually leads to Vata-type diseases. Both under-nourishment and over-nourishment predispose one to weakness of the physical and/or mental digestive fire, thus leading to the production of Digestive Toxins (ama, literally meaning "raw, uncooked, unripened"). Digestive Toxin is a generic term for food (or thought) which is absorbed into the system without having first been properly digested. Such partly-digested material cannot be used by the system, clogs it and creates a toxic reaction.

The usual process by which disease due to excess "wetness" develops is known as "Obstruction to the Pathways" and involves the plugging of some of the channels of body and mind by Digestive Toxins thus preventing Vata from moving in its normal direction. This "angers" or disturbs Vata, causing it to move abnormally through the organism, oft dragging Pitta or Vata along, until it finds a weak point. There the Doshas accumulate, disordering the system and creating a specific disease. The symptoms of such diseases often differ from the symptoms of aggravated Vata because Vata accepts the qualities of whatever it transports. When Vata increases under "dry" conditions, as when the body becomes emaciated or when a hollow organ remains empty for too long, Digestive Toxins are not much involved and the disease produced is usually due mainly to Vata excess alone.

Disruption of Vata's natural direction or rhythm occurs in all diseases. Under the influence of a misdirected Vata the Doshas may move up, down or sideways. The rishi Sharngadhara, paraphrasing Charaka concurs:

"Pitta is lame, Kapha is lame, the tissues and wastes are lame; like the clouds these shower wherever the wind (Vata) carries them." Every disease follows its own path along one or more of the three disease pathways representing deepening penetration of the disease process into the system. These three are the Internal or Visceral Pathway, External or Peripheral Pathway, and Medial or Marma Pathway. The Internal Pathway, which is the digestive tract and the tissue Sap, is usually the first to be affected by the Doshas, which naturally concentrate in the major digestive organs. If the Doshas are not adequately dealt with at this stage they will begin to flow into instead of out of the body, entering the Peripheral Pathway consisting of the other six tissues. If the imbalance is then further suppressed then the toxins and/or the Doshas dive deeper into the tissues and enter the Medial Pathway, which contains all the essential organs. Disease manifestation generally tends to confine itself to a single Pathway at a time; but if more than one Pathway becomes embroiled, treatment becomes much more difficult.

9
Diagnosis

*I*n Ayurveda the diagnostic tests investigate a person's "state," the pattern of movement of tissues, wastes, and Doshas in the body and mind. Your present state reflects your past activities and indicates the direction in which you are moving. Ayurvedic diagnosis begins with an examination of what is right with you, namely how well-nourished, perfectly toned or "excellent" your tissues are. A ruddy complexion, well-formed flesh and fat, solid bones, strong nervous system, and skin and eyes full of luster indicate that the tissues are well-nourished and full of healthy Sap. Only after these "excellences" have been inventoried does one begin the search for deficiencies.

Direct perception is the best way in which to discern a patient's state, though it is sometimes unreliable due to defects of perception. Whatever cannot be known directly must be elicited through three other methods: logical inference, analogy, and the testimony of experts. Seeing, feeling and hearing are the three main methods of direct perception, especially with regard to feces, urine, pulse, tongue and face. Some doctors question their patients closely, while others ask only a few questions. Each physician develops a diagnostic technique in conformity with his or her own constitution.

Physical symptoms are then correlated to the particular Dosha responsible. Excess of Kapha causes mucus and its other vehicles to accumulate within the body, creating obstructive conditions, viz. indigestion, lethargy, cough and nausea. Insufficient Kapha leads to problems like weakness, dryness of skin and mouth, body ache, palpitations and insomnia. Even proper amount of Kapha may accumulate if some obstruction prevents its excretion. Over-production of Pitta generates excess bile and the like, creating such ailments as anger, acidity, increased body heat, burning sensations, yellowness of body and mind, diminished sleep, and excessive hunger and thirst. Obstructed Pitta may also cause these and other varied problems, while insufficient Pitta accounts for signs of coldness, lack of vigor and joy, stiffness, loss of lustre, and weakened digestion. Excess Vata promotes weakness, emaciation, dryness, flatulence, constipation, pain, insomnia, tremors and tics, giddiness, and impairment of sensory and motor functions, whereas decreased Vata reduces metabolism and disturbs the digestion.

As mentioned earlier, an organism's state of health is characterized by the rhythm or gait of Vata. Pulse diagnosis is the method of choice for an examination of these gaits. The radial pulse is examined first, and in some cases other arteries (the carotids or the dorsalis pedis in particular) may also be selected for further examination. Traditionally a man's right arm and a woman's left arm are selected for examination, with the examiner's index finger placed closest to the wrist and the ring finger placed farthest away from the wrist. The index finger reads the condition of the patient's Vata, while the middle finger reads Pitta, and the ring finger Kapha. Because none of the major texts provide specifics of pulse-diagnostic methods, most practitioners evolve their own system, and some use pulse primarily to examine the condition of specific organs.

It is however more common to investigate the pulse's pace, or gait. The pulse-gait in Vata disturbance, for example, often resembles that of a snake or leech as it slithers underneath the skin. Pitta disturbed pulse tends to hop like crows or frogs, and the pulse-gait in a Kapha prone disturbance resembles the swimming movement of a swan. Each disease has its own gait and rhythm; so long as your organism is "possessed" by a disease your energy will move according to its whims. The strength and direction of the disease's gait indicates the length and strength of its existence.

Investigation of both the beginning (the tongue) and the end (the feces and urine) of the alimentary canal is used to gain information on the level of the body's toxicity and on the condition of the doshas in the digestive tract. The first one-third of the tongue represents the area of the body that is governed by Kapha (primarily the chest and head), the middle one-third represents the area that Pitta rules (the area between the diaphragm and the navel), and the back one-third stands for Vata's region (that which is below the navel). No major Ayurvedic text details the locations of the various organ reflexes on the tongue; however, at least one oral tradition of organ-mapping does exist. According to this tradition, the tongue's tip represents the throat, the tongue's root represents the perineum, and all body structures between the throat and perineum are projected onto the tongue's body. Examination of feces predominantly consists of the color, consistency, odor, and presence or absence of undigested food. The color, relative heat or cold, and froth or lack thereof of the urine also reflects body's condition; in particular, the way a drop of oil spreads when dropped onto the surface of the urine indicates which dosha currently predominates.

These and other techniques provide the physician with diagnostic as well as prognostic information on the patient. To know an individual's condition is only half the story; the other half is to know how easy it will be to rectify that condition, and how much of the patient's previous vitality can in fact be restored. Diseases are categorized as easily curable, curable with difficulty, ameliorable (the disease remains under control only so

long as treatment goes on) or incurable. In an incurable condition excessive measures to prolong life are not commonly employed, nor an immi-
nent demise predicted. Instead, the patient is made comfortable and is encouraged to prepare for eventual death, for Ayurveda regards a good death
as being the consummation of a good life.

10

Treatment

*D*iseases manifest due to the impact of many causes at an opportune time and place, and they disappear by change of time or place or by withdrawal of their causes. The essence of treatment is removal of the cause. Diseases mainly due to physical causes require "scientific" therapy (the use of herbs, diet, manipulation, and so on). Those mainly due to psychological disturbance require "conquest of the mind," necessitating restraint of the mind from the desire for unwholesome objects. And diseases of the spirit need "divine" therapy, spiritual rituals and penances. Since "crimes against wisdom" motivated by desire are the ultimate causes of disease, the elimination of desire is the ultimate treatment for disease. Desire is however difficult to extirpate from the mind. Ayurveda has therefore established methods by which desire can be disciplined; through beneficial routines to maintain proper functioning of the organism during health and by therapeutic procedures coupled with diet and lifestyle changes during sickness in order to return the wandering Doshas to their proper bodily paths and the individual to his or her proper life path.

Any substance and any activity in the world can be and has been used therapeutically in Ayurveda. Generally, however, medical intervention used at the physical level is of four types: diet, activity, purification, and palliation. Accumulation of the Doshas should be treated with changes in diet and activity; when they become aggravated, palliating or pacifying them with substances of opposite qualities is best. Once the Doshas escape their reservoir organs it is best to remove them from the system; if this is impossible they must be neutralized with medicine. Localized treatment is always beneficial to that weak part of the body in which the Doshas localize. Since dietary indiscretion is the most common cause in the majority of diseases, changes in diet are often the single most important aspect of therapy.

Whenever feasible Ayurveda always favors gradual over instantaneous cures to prevent unnecessary shocks to the system. Gradual elimination of addictions is less disrupting to your internal balance than is the immediate, "cold turkey" procedure. Since an organism always needs time to acclimatize itself to its new state, medical treatment too, should never be stopped abruptly.

As each individual is unique, each patient requires a different treatment program. In as much as all physical diseases are caused, either directly or indirectly by Dosha imbalance, all treatment is based fundamentally on the treatment of the Doshas. When Digestive Toxins are present in the digestive tract, treatment usually begins with a near-total fast of one to two days to digest and remove the accumulated toxins and to prepare the body for purification.

The Doshas are actively excreted from the body by Five Purifications (panchakarma): emesis (therapeutic vomiting), purgation, enema, nasal medication, and bloodletting. Before any form of purification is performed, the Dosha to be eliminated must be made to leave the tissues to which it has strayed, and return to its reservoir organs in the digestive tract. This "change of Dosha direction" is usually done by applying medicated oils to the body and thus inducing it to sweat. Once a Dosha has returned back to its reservoir organ, substances are administered to encourage it to increase its force there. For example, before emesis, which is often used to relieve Kapha, some doctors increase Kapha by giving the patient a mixture of yogurt, molasses and salt. Only then is vomiting induced. Similar procedures are followed for the other Doshas.

Emesis (therapeutic vomiting) is the main purification method for Kapha, though purgation may also be used. Emesis is a strong purification technique as it removes mucus and other undesirable substances from the stomach, chest and other locations where Kapha concentrates, and encourages an upward flow of energy in contrast to Kapha's normal heavy, downward movement. In contrast purification for Vata should be mild so as to restrain its normally intense nature. The purification of choice for Vata is enema because it helps Vata's downward movement (being Airy it tends to flow upward), and does not remove much material from the body (as Vata people tend to lack physical substance). Besides it does not weaken the digestive fire as emesis and purgation do. Purgation and bloodletting are preferred purification techniques for the removal of excess Pitta because it concentrates in the digestive tract and in the blood with its inherent heat. Emesis is also employed sometimes for Pitta if it is trying to escape the body by moving upward (causing such symptoms as nausea and heartburn).

Purification is only administered, however, if the patient is relatively strong and the disease is relatively weak. In other cases, and during childhood, old age, pregnancy, and other such circumstances palliation of the Doshas alone is performed. Palliation is a seven-step procedure which includes medicine to digest toxins, medicine to increase the digestive fire, appropriate diet and drinks, exercise, sunbathing, and exposure to fresh-air, each prescribed according to the patient's requirements. Ayurvedic medicines are prepared from a wide variety of substances derived from animal, vegetable and mineral sources and produced in the forms of medicated pills, powders, jams, wines, milks, ghees (clarified butter) and oils.

Each Dosha requires a unique therapeutic strategy for the restoration of internal balance. Specifically, Vata's main remedies are heat and oil, externally and internally, because they counteract its dry and cold qualities. Salty taste works best in small amounts both in medicine and food, since it improves appetite and digestion, and is antispasmodic and slightly laxative. Only thereafter sour and sweet tastes are considered and employed. Medicinal wines are beneficial, as are medicines which have been potentiated one hundred or one thousand times. Massage of all kinds is very desirable. In certain cases shock treatments, "de-memorizing therapy" (something like "de-programming"), and binding are used. The patient's anxieties should be eliminated, and he or she should be furnished plenty of entertainment and total relaxation to promote a free flow of Prana in the channels of body and mind.

Pitta, naturally needs to be cooled. Bitter taste performs this best, followed by sweet and astringent. Sweet-smelling scents (perfumes, incense, flowers) help to overcome Pitta's strong odor. Especially efficacious are sandalwood, lotus and rose, all of which provide a cooling effect as well. Cool showers, moon-bathing, pearl necklaces, white clothes, and sojourn in green gardens amid fountains are other means to calm the system. When Pitta is permitted to increase, it inflames the body's tissues thus interrupting the flow of Prana in the channels. This can be ameliorated by reducing Pitta's native intensity with soothing music and by meditation to quieten the mind. Regular consumption of raw food and a job or hobby of an absorbing nature are other routines that should be followed for a timely recovery.

Kapha requires intensity and activity to break up its natural inertia and lethargy. The pungent taste, composed as it is of the Fire and Air Elements, is the best Kapha-controlling taste, followed by bitter and astringent. When toxins are present, bitter should first be utilized to clear the channels before pungent things are employed to reawaken the digestive fire. The astringent taste is utilized if excess "moisture" removal is required. All medicines and foods should be hot, intense and dry. Aged wines and liqueurs in small doses, nights without sleep, frequent sexual intercourse, vigorous exercise like wrestling, running and jumping to cause copious sweating, fasting, smoking, rough dry warm clothes, and extremely hot baths all decrease Kapha. Saddling Kapha patients with responsibilities and preventing them from indulging in their normal stupor helps to overcome their internal stagnation.

The typical Ayurvedic treatment consists of a remedy, a vehicle, and a diet regimen. While remedies are most commonly administered either through mouth or through anus (i.e. by enema), those that target structures in the throat and head are frequently administered through the nostrils. Pastes and oils are usually applied locally, though in certain conditions whole-body application is used to exert a systemic effect. The vehicle helps the remedy by proper digestion and absorption, and catalyzes its effect so as to reduce the dose and thus prevent possible side-effects. While hot water can be used as a vehicle for almost all preparations, other common vehicles include honey, ghee, oil, jams, and wines.

Most substances used as medicines can be employed singly or in combination, the choice depending primarily on the physician's preference. Single drugs possess the virtue of simplicity, while compounds are usually formulated from several substances which share specific therapeutic qualities and so synergize with each other. Since most medicaments can affect the body in more than one way, specific vehicles are prescribed to help target the medicine.

The way in which substances are prepared for administration depends on the purpose for which they are to be used. For example, aloe vera is used in powdered form to purify the uterus or the digestive tract, in crude form as the juice to soothe burns or ulcers, and as a medicinal wine for liver disorders. Sometimes the preparation of the substance is limited by its nature, i.e. while it is easy to obtain juice from a pulpy leaf like aloe it may be almost impossible to do so from more fibrous leaves, which will have to be powdered, decocted, or otherwise extracted. The nature of the Dosha involved also affects formulation: Kapha conditions often do better with dried powders, Vata problems with medicated oils and medicinal wines, and Pitta disturbances with fresh juices and medicated ghees (see illustration 17).

Minerals need to be purified as well as "humanized" before they become fit for consumption by human beings. Most minerals are transformed into bhasma (literally, "ash"); these "ashes" are prepared by incinerating the mineral in the presence of specific herbal or animal substances. The average mineral must be incinerated at least seven times before it can be administered, but since each incineration potentiates the mineral's activity, a larger number of incinerations is almost always desirable. Mica, for example, works best after being potentiated one thousand times.

By astute purification and palliation a physician removes all obstructions to the free movement of Prana so that Prana can again inflame the digestive fire, thus reviving the patient's immunity. It is impossible to be healthy until the life force has free access to all parts of the body. The seers who cognized Ayurveda did so for the benefit of "dwellers in cities and towns." They realized that urbanites become more prone to disease because of the combination of various factors of environmental pollution and due to overcrowding. Such people may become candidates for two therapies which are unique to Ayurveda: rejuvenation (rasayana) and virilization (bajikarana). Virilization is meant to enhance fertility, and rejuvenation to prevent future diseases by enhancing immunity. These, like Ayurveda's other therapeutic modalities aim to maximize harmony between the external and the internal environment of the individual.

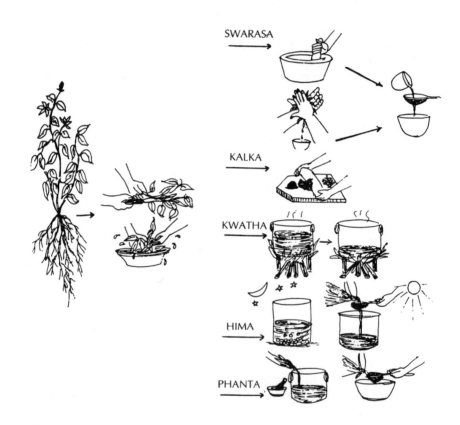

SWARASA

KALKA

KWATHA

HIMA

PHANTA

17. Five Types of Ayurvedic Preparations

According to Ayurvedic pharmacology there are five main methods for preparing medicines: expressed juice (swarasa), pulvis (kalka), decoction (kwatha), cold infusion (hima) amd hot infusion (phanta).

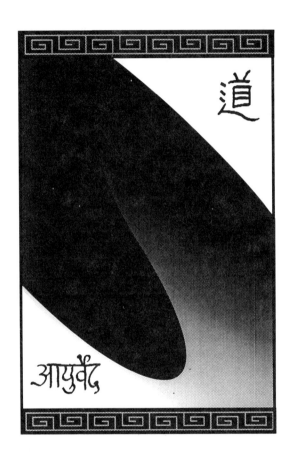

PART THREE
TRADITIONS IN COMPARISON

1
Historical Considerations

*B*oth Indian and Chinese medicine are unique systems that arose independently, remaining intimately associated with their own indigenous religious and cultural perspectives. This, however, did not hinder the exchange of information and absorption of concepts and practices from one system to the other, or from other surrounding cultures. Tracing the exact routing and giving concrete dates to these transmissions of knowledge is extremely difficult, but certain general themes may nevertheless be inferred from the mass of information available.

An important historical event occurred sometime during the third or fourth century B.C. that clearly establishes that these two societies were indeed in communication with each other. At that time India already possessed a highly evolved literary society which had produced scores of texts on such topics as religion, astrology and medicine. The preeminent Ayurvedic text *Charaka Samhita* was already many hundred years old, while the landmark *Yellow Emperor's Inner Classic* was only then being compiled in China. During this period reports started to circulate in China about soma, the psychotropic plant associated with mystical experiences which had occupied an important place in early Indian religion. In the Indian context the use of soma is known to have played a central role in the *Rig Veda*, a scripture that appeared prior to 1000 B.C.

Soma was promoted in China as possessing the power to bestow immortality, and the persistent and enticing reports eventually led Emperor Qin Shi (reigned 221-207 B.C.), first Emperor of a unified China, to order the procurement of this wondrous plant. Eventually, the Emperor himself went to the western mountains in an unsuccessful search. Despite this failure, the Emperor refused to give up, and apparently gave permission and support to a peculiar man named Su Fu, who was sent with a large contingent of virginal children on a sea voyage to bring back this divine substance. The first journey did not go well, and on Su Fu's return, he was re-equipped and sent off again, but nothing more is known about this later mission.

The Chinese never did obtain soma, even though continuous efforts were made during the Han Dynasty (206 B.C.-220 A.D.), and even today no one knows soma's true identity, despite much search and speculation. This should not be surprising since according to Tantric tradition, there is no one "soma". Many different substances can be used as soma, if they are employed in the proper way at the proper time. This deep interest by the Chinese in soma did at least stimulate, and perhaps initiate the development of the Taoist alchemical arts. A momentous spin-off was an enthusiastic research into China's own plants and minerals as well as the systemization of Internal Medicine. Clearly the mysterious soma kindled the interest of the Chinese in the lands to the west.

Other evidence suggests that there had been contacts between these two ancient Asian cultures before the 4th century B.C. There are for example some remarkable similarities between their ancient systems of astrology, including the division of the sky into twenty-eight (later twenty-seven) lunar mansions (Sanskrit nakshatra, Chinese xiu) comprised of similar star groupings. The original purpose of these divisions is not known, though most likely they were used to keep track of the moon, which moves along the ecliptic about thirteen degrees per day, about the width of one lunar mansion. Nine of the twenty-eight nakshatra stars were also used by the Chinese to determine the twenty-eight xiu, and eleven more are in the same constellation as other xiu stars. Both systems have stars in common—ten in the case of the nakshatras—with the set of thirty-six used by the Babylonians, suggesting at least the possibility that both systems had been enriched by Mesopotamian astrological knowledge early on.

The ancient philosophy of China prior to 4th century B.C. was of course the Yin-Yang doctrine, based on an image of a harmonic polarity found in all nature. In India however, ancient philosophy emphasized triune doctrines. A primary concept was that of the Three Attributes (gunas) or propensities within phenomena towards activity (rajas), inertia (tamas) and equilibrium (sattva). This concept pervades religious belief as well, and the three chief gods of India represent the fundamental powers in the universe: Brahma, the Creator, is the embodiment of Rajas; Shiva, the Destroyer, embodies Tamas; and Vishnu, the Preserver, balances the other two. While we can view the dynamic dualism of Yin and Yang as embodying the tendencies toward inertia and activity respectively, the Indian concept of equilibrium, a neutral reconciling force between positive and negative, is lacking in the Chinese model. For the Chinese, the space between Yin and Yang was occupied by a creative tension that materially manifests in the form of Qi.

Within the Indian sciences there was, very early on, a highly developed theory of the Five Elements (pancha mahabhutas). By comparison, before the fourth century B.C., an archaic concept of five fundamental substances did exist in China, but the importance of this idea was far eclipsed by the Yin-Yang doctrine. According to historians it was Zou Yin (359-270 B.C.) who developed and integrated a unique version of the Five Elements (wu xing) into the mainstream of Chinese science and religion. There is a reasonable probability that the impetus for development of the

Chinese Five-Element doctrine, as first expounded by Zou Yin, may have come from the Indian theory, though the Chinese modified and integrated this foreign concept to suit their own world view. In fact vast differences evolved between these fundamental concepts, as can be seen on the most cursory level by the similarity of only three component Elements within each system.

Essentially, the Indian concept of the Five Elements evolved from a hierarchical mode of thinking that underlines most ancient Hindu sciences and philosophies, an approach which is sometimes called "essence extraction." The Five Elements are viewed as emerging each from its precursor in a chain of causation from Ether through Earth. In this model each element contains representative parts of the other four elements, but the element in question predominates. The Earth Element, for example, is thus an "essence" of Earth, a concentration of Earthiness manifesting within the context of the whole Group of Five. Because of its relative predominance it prevents the other Elements from exerting their influences significantly.

In contrast to the relatively static portrayal of the Elements in Ayurveda, the Chinese with no hierarchical order emphasized instead the dynamic inter-relationships which exist among the Five Elements. Chinese theory is dynamic within the relatively static context of embodied life, and does not seek to connect the Elements to their ultimate source in the Absolute; Ayurvedic theory is static, relatively speaking, within the dynamic context of the perpetual projection of consciousness into matter and its equally continuous withdrawal therefrom.

In each society prevailing philosophical beliefs contributed greatly to the development of their medical systems, especially Taoism in China and the Yoga philosophy in India. Although various forms of Yoga had been practiced in India since prehistoric times, it was left for Patanjali (circa 3rd century B.C.) to integrate it with the Sankhya philosophy and to organize it into a coherent system. The Taoist and Sankhya philosophies have much in common: they both propose an original formless non-manifest primordial source (purusha/wu) and a creative force or potential which initiated the cosmic process of differentiation (prakruti/tai yi). Further divergence of the cosmos arose due to primal tendencies (gunas/yin-yang) arising from this creative potential, and the Five Elements (pancha mahabhutas/wu xing) are essential manifestations of this diversity. Another vital concept shared by the Taoist and Samkhya philosophies is the view that all things have their own unique nature (prakriti/de).

Historically, the era of the Han Dynasty was a period of an outward focus for China. By 138 B.C. the Silk Road to the west and the Burma Road (115 B.C.) to the south had opened up commerce and exchange of ideas and technology with foreign lands. On China's western frontier beyond the Kunlun Mountains a southward branch of the Silk Road led to India. China also embarked on great navigational explorations to open up sea links to the south and east. By the 2nd century B.C., boats from imperial China had reached far shores in the Indian Ocean, reportedly to present day Sri Lanka, at the time when Indian civilization and religion were rapidly spreading.

The arrival of Ayurveda accompanied Sri Lanka's conversion to Buddhism by Mahinda, the brother of King Ashoka, the enlightened ruler of the Maurya empire of northern India. King Ashoka, who after a long and bloody campaign to capture the Kingdom of Kalinga felt great remorse at all the slaughter, converted to Buddhism in 260 B.C. and renounced foreign aggression. After conversion, he sent out emissaries to all the neighboring lands, and possibly to more distant realms such as Greece and China, to spread his new-found beliefs. Hindu invasions of Sri Lanka began perhaps as early as the second century B.C., and by 100 A.D. Hinduization of the Malay peninsula, Indochina and the islands of present day western Indonesia had successfully begun.

Indeed, along with religion and culture, Ayurvedic concepts and practices spread throughout South-East Asia. In Cambodia, for example, Sanskrit inscriptions of Ayurvedic doctrines and quotations from Sushruta's treatise dating back to the ninth century A.D. can still be found carved on stone. Another example of Ayurveda's influence in this region is the incorporation of the Nadis and Marma theory into Thai massage, and practiced even to this day.

This period of outward expansion and external focus of both cultures also favored the introduction of Buddhism from its native Indian soil into China. Indeed by 100 A.D. already there were many regional strongholds of Buddhism in China. The Buddhist monks Kasyapa, Matanga and Dharmaraksa carried the gospel of Buddha to the imperial Chinese court from India sometime during the 1st century A.D., and the first Buddhist texts from Sanskrit and Pali translated into Chinese are known to have been written then. The introduction of Buddhism, naturally due to Buddhist belief in compassion and removal of suffering, also led to the propagation of effective medical care. Buddhist medical concepts incorporated the Ayurvedic model, but expanded and emphasized the spiritual causes and treatment of illness as well.

An interesting figure of this period was Hua Tuo (110- 208 A.D.) who is revered as a brilliant physician and surgeon, and also as the originator of various Taoist physical exercises (tao yin), especially the system based on the movements of five animals. Reports on his surgical techniques bear striking resemblance to the surgical methods expounded in Ayurvedic texts, in particular the usage of a concoction of hemp (ma fei san) to engender an analgesic effect in the patient prior to the operation. Circumstantial evidence strongly indicates that Hua Tuo in all probability learnt at least some of his skills from Indian sources (see illustration 18).

India, whose written tradition of surgery begins with the *Sushruta Samhita* (perhaps 600 B.C.), has had a longer and more sustained surgical

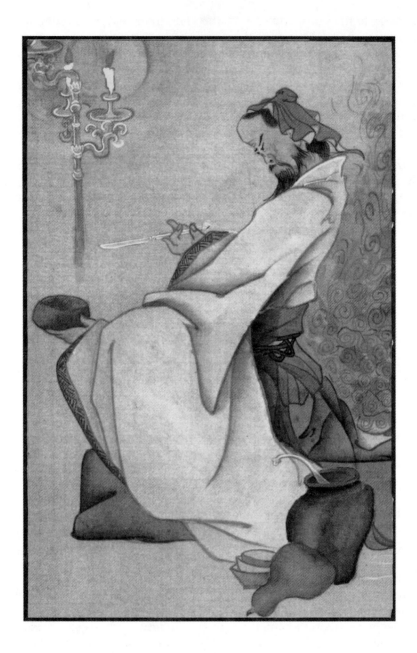

18. Hua Tuo

A contemporary drawing of the much revered master physician and surgeon Hua Tuo who lived during the Eastern Han Dynasty (25-200 A.D.). Here he is depicted patiently preparing one of his medicinal formulas, many of which are still being used in China today.

tradition than China. In this text the use of hemp decoctions for surgical analgesia is clearly mentioned. Indeed, India has a long tradition of using hemp in medicine. The gifted 5th century B.C. physician and surgeon Jivaka, attended on the Buddha himself. He was also a patron of the medical arts and sciences to the Buddhists in India, as was Hua Tuo to the Chinese. A few centuries later, even the removal of cataracts by surgery seems to have been introduced into China from India.

With the growth and influence of Buddhism both in India and China a great deal of religious, cultural and medical interchange took place. Many Indian monks transversed the frontier regions of India to spread Buddhist teachings into the adjoining kingdoms. By the 3rd century A.D., Chinese monks and scholars, too, started to journey to the land of Buddha's birth in search of knowledge. The first well-documented Chinese pilgrim during this early period of exchange was Fa Xian (337-422 A.D.) who went overland to India. Fa Xian studied for 14 years in the Buddhist lands of South Asia, including Sri Lanka, before returning to China via the by then well established southern sea route.

The golden age of Buddhism in Asia coincides with the glorious period of Ayurveda in India and of Chinese Medicine in China approximately from the 4th to 10th century A.D. During this period Buddhism found popular appeal, and at times official sanction, promoting closer relationships between various Buddhist kingdoms in Asia. However, Buddhism did not completely supplant either Hinduism in India or Taoist-Confucian teachings in China. This period saw intense development in all sciences and brought significant social changes, especially during the time of the Gupta Empires (4th to 6th centuries A.D.) in India and the Six Dynasties period (3rd to 7th centuries A.D.) in China.

One important Buddhist sage of South Indian origin, Boddhidharma (479-543 A.D.), traveled by ship to China in the beginning of the 6th century A.D. and originated a new religious community. After spending some time at the imperial court in Nanjing he continued his journey until he reached the Sungshan Mountains where he founded the Shaolin monastery. The unique meditative practices taught by him there are considered to be the origin of the Chan (Zen in Japanese) school, and therefore he is recognized as the first patriarch of one of the extent preeminent systems of philosophy and spiritual disciplines. Boddhidharma also introduced a form of martial arts (shaolin kung fu) that has become famous the world over in modern times. The scholars generally believe that what this sage had actually introduced was kalarippayattu, the South Indian martial art from the state of Kerala, but as usual it underwent a thorough transformation into a characteristically Chinese form (see illustration 19).

Buddhist doctrine was also subject to such transmutation; for example, the masculine figure of Avalokitesvara, the Boddhisattva of Divine Compassion who plays a significant role in the healing arts, had by the

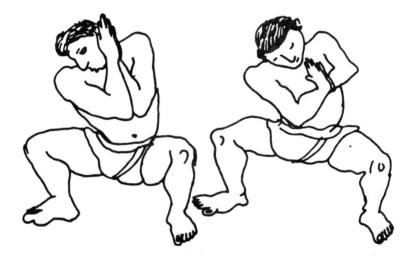

19. Kalarippayatu

The figures reveal two typical preparatory moves in the South Indian martial arts tradition of kalarippayatu. Masters of this tradition are not only renowned for their combative abilities but often for their healing skills and spiritual attainment.

7th century A.D. been transformed into Guan Yin, the Goddess of Mercy, a distinctly feminine figure.

In China, Buddhist medical teachings emphasized the Indian concepts of the Elements, although Buddhists refer usually to a four Element system, the five Great Elements of Ayurveda minus Ether (akasha). It is possible that the Buddhist concept reflects a Hellenistic influence, but deducing correspondences by number alone can be misleading. In India, for example, the venerable Sushruta advocated a four Dosha concept. He included blood as one of the doshas because of the importance of blood to a surgeon. It is also known that Hellenistic medicine borrowed heavily from India through the writings of Pythagoras (circa 6th century B.C.) the philosopher and inventor, who, it is known, had journeyed to India and later had such a significant influence on the Hippocratic school.

Efforts were indeed made in China to reconcile the Buddhist-Ayurvedic concept of the Elements with the doctrines of Chinese Medicine. The Indian teachings referred to the great Elements as generating and differentiating the human body's various tissues, while the Five Chinese Elements envisioned more the functional relationships between processes. The Ayurvedic concept of Three Doshas, however, presented a difficult challenge for reconciliation from the Chinese viewpoint, and it was never really incorporated into the Chinese paradigm, mainly due to the strangeness of the concept and the difficulty translators had in finding adequate terms. Various Buddhist scriptures from the 2nd century A.D. onward, in fact, reveal great inconsistency in their translations of Ayurvedic terms and doctrines. For example, the term Dosha was translated into Chinese as poison (tu) or at other times into grave illnesses (da ping) which only vaguely convey its original connotation as a fundamental fault; nor does either term reflect the basic concept that the doshas actually arise from and are a condensed form of the Five Elements. And the individual Doshas were translated into the terms wind for Vata, heat for Pitta and cold for Kapha. Such superficial translation of the Doshas inadequately denotes their unique individual attributes and erroneously links them to three of the Chinese medical concepts of the six exogenous Pernicious Influences.

The celebrated physician of the Tang Dynasty, Sun Simiao (581-682 A.D.), a devoted Buddhist, tried in his writings to reconcile these two medical traditions. He wrote on a wide field of medical topics including alchemy, bone setting, Buddhist spirituality and etiology based on karma, states and treatment of possession, acupuncture and botanical medicine. But, in general, even in Sun Simiao's exposition a genuine understanding of the theoretical concepts of Indian medicine was lacking, and only some comparatively minor elements were eventually incorporated into Chinese medicine.

China in turn had a lot to offer to India in terms of theory and practical medicine. In this context Yi Xing (635-731 A.D.), a Chinese Buddhist monk who studied in India at Nalanda University between the years 671-695 A.D. and who thus had a good insight into both systems of medicine, has remarked that ". . . in the healing arts of acupuncture, moxibustion and in diagnosis through pulse, China has never been superseded by any country of Jambudvipa (India)." Yi Xing also observed many beneficial practices in India including the usage of therapeutic fasting that were different from those of his native land. But for some obscure reason, the useful Chinese techniques of acupuncture did not seem to have left a great impression on Ayurvedic and Buddhist medicine, for no records point to its adoption in India. Yi Xing is said to have brought more than 400 Buddhist texts back with him to China; of which 56 he translated into Chinese himself. In recording his own journey, he also included biographies of a large number of Chinese monks who were traveling to India mainly by the sea route.

In spite of the seeming lack of interest in Chinese acupuncture among Buddhists in India there appears to have existed in Sri Lanka an indigenous form of acupuncture. Even in present day Sri Lanka one comes across reports of acupuncture being used by traditional healers in cases of snake bite, and the use of acupressure on elephants! Dr. A. Jayasuria suggests that this unique system of acupuncture was a branch of Deshiya Vedakamae, an ancient medical system practiced on that island well before the arrival of Ayurvedic medicine during the middle of the 3rd century B.C. This does not however preclude the possibility of Chinese acupuncture having influenced the development of this healing science in Sri Lanka, since contact between these two lands did exist as far back as the 2nd century B.C.

The Sri Lankan system of acupuncture utilized a large number of therapeutic points (nilas, meaning command point) along with a large number of forbidden points that closely resemble the present day concept of the Marmas in Ayurveda. In contrast to the Chinese system, however, a unique feature of Sri Lankan acupuncture is the absence of any concept of Meridians (jingluo). In Sri Lanka the utilization of acupuncture in veterinary medicine seems to have been practiced to a much greater extent than even in China, and ancient charts have been found illustrating the points for use in treating, among others, elephants, water buffalo, tigers and pigs. King Buddhadasa (reigned 337-365 A.D.) has been reported to be a well-versed surgeon and acupuncturist himself who treated both human beings and animals alike.

Tibetan medicine clearly shows the impact of both Ayurveda and Chinese medicine. Ayurveda entered Tibet in the wake of Buddhism around 6th century A.D., and still remains at the core of Tibetan medicine. King Srongtsan Gampo, who reigned in the first half of the 7th century A.D., was responsible for opening Tibet's doors to new cultural and religious influences from the surrounding kingdoms. It was during this period that even the Tibetan alphabet was adopted from Sanskrit. The king was so keen on the study of medicine that he had a medical conference organized inviting doctors from India, Persia and China. It was recorded at that time that each representative translated into Tibetan a medical work from their respective country.

Over the ensuing centuries Tibetan doctors acquired further texts and knowledge from neighboring lands, and today Tibetan written medical tradition is a repository for many classical Ayurvedic texts that have become extinct in their native India. Even the most important text in Tibetan medicine, the *Four Tantras* (*Gyushi*) is considered to be of Indian origin. Buddhist legend says that Jivaka, the Buddha's physician actually wrote down these medical teachings which over the centuries were supplemented by writings of other distinguished Indian and Tibetan doctors.

Tibetans acknowledge the influence of Chinese medicine in the practices of acupuncture, the system of pulse diagnosis and inspection of the tongue. Pulse diagnosis (nadi pariksha) makes its appearance in mainstream Ayurvedic literature only during the 12th century A.D., with the Sharngadhara Samhita. India's system of pulse diagnosis in all probability came from the Muslim medical system of Unani Tibbia or from Tibetan, both of which may have originally acquired this knowledge of the pulse from the Chinese. Tibet's great contribution to Ayurveda has been the detailed development of urine analysis (mutra pariksha).

Tibetan medicine had also developed a rather sophisticated knowledge of anatomy, which was acquired from their long-standing experience with human dissection. Tibetans, out of necessity, had long ago adopted the practice of "celestial burial" because of their country's harsh terrain in which the ground is frozen for extended periods during the year and the scarcity of wood for cremation. This form of so-called burial, still widely practiced, proceeds with the ritual dissection of the deceased, and then followed by the feeding of the parts to vultures on the hill tops. Over time this anatomical knowledge found its way into Ayurveda and to a lesser extent into China. Indeed, Tibet was the site of two well known Buddhist medical centers (Chogpori and Menchikhang), between the twelfth to sixteenth century A.D., where monks came to study even from foreign countries.

During the golden age of Buddhism, many techniques and other practical aspects of medicine were exchanged between China and India, and one area in which this is certainly evident is in medicinal pharmacology. China imported hemp, sandalwood, cardamom, long pepper, camphor, calamus root, datura and cinnamon from India, while India obtained rhubarb, sarsaparilla, angelica, licorice, ginseng, mugwort and tea from China. The exchange of ideas stimulated each other's understanding of the pharmacodynamics of plants and minerals, and ushered in new advancements in the preparation of these plant/mineral based medicines (see illustration 20).

Arabic frankincense   Mongolian garlic   Chinese quince

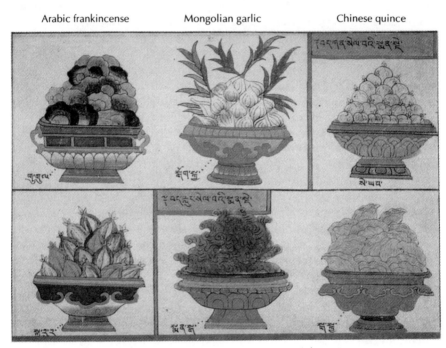

Indian embelic myrobalan   Tibetan ginger   South Chinese kaempteris galanga

20. Medicinal Substances from the *Blue Beryl*

These six medicinal substances were in common use in Tibet when they appeared in the *Blue Beryl* Treatise of Sangye Gyamtso (1653-1705 A.D.) As shown from *left to right top row*: Arabic frankincense, Mongolian garlic, and Chinese quince, (*bottom row*) Indian embelic myrobalan, Tibetan ginger and South Chinese kaempteria galanga. Numerous medicinal plants and minerals, including those represented above, were traded throughout Asia.

The alchemical schools of both countries were predominantly responsible for the exchange of this knowledge. These schools in those days were intimately linked to the religious institutions of Taoism and Tantra, and to a lesser extent Buddhism. Historically the Chinese had a more highly advanced knowledge of the alchemical arts since the times of the Han Dynasty, and they are credited with considerably aiding the advancement of Indian alchemy. The earliest adept at alchemy known to have traveled between the two countries was Siddha Bogar, a famous Chinese alchemist, who during the 3rd century A.D. journeyed, taught and eventually settled in what is now Tamil Nadu in southern India. Legend has it that Bogar also returned briefly to China with a group of Indian disciples before settling back in Tamilnad. Unlike most Chinese travelers to India, however, Bogar was apparently a Taoist rather than a Buddhist.

Alchemy has two forms of expression: an outward search, dealing with the transformation of substances for the benefit of the adept, and an inward quest, dealing with special internal practices for personal transformation. External alchemy stimulated intense research into plants and minerals, generating new knowledge that was imbibed into such diverse fields as medicine, metallurgic sciences, botany or even in warfare (as with the discovery of gunpowder). Initially gunpowder, literally a "fire drug" (huoyao), was a product of alchemical experimentation that was subsequently used as a medicine to cure skin diseases. In general, mineral substances have a most important role to play in external alchemy with mercury and sulfur being the two most significant.

It is a curious fact that in China mercury denotes the female principle and sulfur the masculine principle, while in India it is just the reverse. Mercury is considered feminine or Yin in Chinese alchemy due to its dissolving and softening effects and its coagulative and liquid form. In contrast Sulfur is considered masculine or Yang on account of its drying and hardening effect, and a solid, rhombic form. Cinnabar contains elements of both mercury and sulfur, thus considered, in Chinese alchemy, the quintessential mineral for purposes of transformation.

In Indian alchemy properly transformed mercury was found to promote the production of semen, while transformed sulfur is used to purify the blood and regulate the menses. It is therefore highly likely that the difference in opinion between the two systems over the gender of these two substances arises mainly from Chinese alchemy's consideration of physical properties to determine gender whereas in India physiological effects seem to have led them to the reverse conclusion. However, Indian alchemy concurs with its Chinese counterpart in accepting cinnabar (mercuric sulfide) as the great transformer, and Ayurveda also makes great use of black sulfide of mercury (mercurous sulfide) mainly in therapeutic preparations.

The internal alchemical practices of Taoism and Tantra are remarkably alike, especially in their vision of the subtle body. Tantra places great emphasis on awakening the energy within the Nadis and Chakras while in Taoism a very similar concept of the Three Fields of Influences (san qi hai dan tian) and the Extraordinary Vessels exists. The unique Indian concept of the Chakras historically is of much greater antiquity and most likely inspired the Taoist version of the Three Fields. In both systems the general idea is to vitalize these structures with energy (prana/qi) to initiate a process of psychophysical and spiritual transformation.

Extensive communication between China and India did not unfortunately last for very long. The first Muslim invasion in the 8th century A.D. blocked travel along the Silk Road. Moreover Buddhism, the religion that had directly spawned the cultural and trade contacts, had already entered into a state of severe decline in India, and would do so in China one century later. No significant trade or cross-cultural activity seems to have occurred during the medieval periods of India and China, and Ayurveda and Chinese medicine were essentially isolated from one another from the 10th century A.D. onward.

Classical Ayurveda began to lose its vitality during this age, though the medical systems of the Siddhas (alchemists) and Muslims flourished, and their thoughts and methods did influence Ayurveda's development. In the China of that era there was a return to Confucianism which coincided with foreign invasions, isolation, and internal divisions within the Middle Kingdom for the next 450 years. Chinese medicine, which had acquired a firm foundation prior to that turbulent era, nevertheless slowly progressed, adding a number of new ideas and innovations to its classical form. Thereafter, however, from about the early part of the Ming Dynasty (1368-1644 A.D.), Chinese medicine entered into a long period of decline. In both these countries the introduction of European medicine, beginning in the 18th century A.D., severely challenged the integrity and influence of their indigenous medical systems. It was only after throwing off the foreign domination that governments of both nations were able to provide meaningful support and sponsorship to these ancient healing traditions.

2
Energetic Physiology

*A*yurveda and Chinese medicine have developed since antiquity an impressive and integral understanding of the human physiological and energetic state. Unfortunately in neither tradition did the in-depth study of anatomy receive an equally high priority. Comparatively, the Indians due to their ancient tradition of surgery derived a greater depth of anatomical knowledge than the Chinese. However both cultures seem to have suffered in this endeavor from the same cause—the objections by the orthodox segment—which led often enough to outright prohibition of the dissection of human cadavers.

In ancient China, dissection was considered profane because it risked disturbing the normal departure of the soul from the body, and so officially sanctioned dissections were generally performed only on criminals after execution. Traditional beliefs such as Confucianism which encouraged ancestor worship were hostile to anyone who disturbed the remains of the departed, for they believed that dissection might interfere with the Yin soul's (Po) return to the earth. Such a soul might then become a wayward ghost, unable to complete its journey after death. Pieces of jade were placed upon the orifices of the deceased bodies of the rich and famous so that the Yin soul would not escape, thus ensuring its return into the earth with the dissolution of the physical elements.

Similar prohibitions were in force in classical India, where rituals were performed after death to ensure that the deceased will enjoy healthy, undeformed limbs and organs in his or her next birth, and any damage to the corpse before its cremation was considered likely to show up on the succeeding incarnation. Additionally, for a high-caste Hindu to touch a corpse was and is considered to be a profound defilement, one which could be counteracted only through intensive and complex purifications. There was also the ever-present awareness of the danger that the dissector might choose to use some of the dissected body parts in black magic rituals. In spite of all these impediments, dissection seems to have been practiced, though probably mainly on the sly, and students augmented their skills by practicing surgery on dummies, melons, dead animals, and lotus stems.

Some materialists have argued that the two systems concentrated on the energetic aspects of physiology because they were prevented from refining their anatomical knowledge, but available evidence suggests that in fact both systems actively valued the vital above the merely physical. Both systems describe the existence of a pervasive life force, called Qi by the Chinese and Prana by the Indians, and the conception of this life force or energy and its functions within the human body including the belief that this substance flows through subtle pathways or Meridians (nadis/ jingluo) appear to be remarkably similar in both systems. Though the Chinese did develop the concept and mapping of the Meridians to a more advanced level mainly from their experience with acupuncture, the Ayurvedic idea of the Marmas also appears to be closely akin to the Chinese concept of an acupuncture point. Also in virtual agreement are the concepts of Blood (rakta/xue) and Essence (ojas/jing) in both systems.

The development of the Meridian theory, by the Chinese, closely parallels their profound knowledge of hydrology, which includes such practices as canal making, irrigation systems and water conservation methods. As far back as the 6th century B.C. many hydrologic projects were undertaken to facilitate China's agricultural development and dependability, as well its inland transportation through shipping. One testament to China's technical mastery of hydrology is the Grand Canal, built about 2,400 years ago and stretching nearly 1,800 kilometers from Beijing in the north to Hangzhou in the south. The Chinese concept of the human Meridian system is decidedly patterned upon the mechanistic model of these ancient hydrologic principles. Examples within the Meridian theory of this hydrologic notion are the concepts of graduated systems of greater to smaller channels in which Qi circulates; the 24 hour circulation of Meridian Qi; the existence of source and connecting points along each Meridian's flow and so on.

According to Chinese medicine the body is composed of five basic substances which provide and maintain life and from which all other tissues are derived. The five primary substances namely Qi, Blood, Fluids, Essence and Spirit are energetic reflections of the Five Elements. The substances have no hierarchical structure: rather these substances are dependent upon and support each other. According to the traditional Chinese viewpoint, other tissues and organs are derived from the matrix of these substances. The Five Elements play an energetic role in linking substances with specific tissues, organs and structures.

By contrast, in the Ayurvedic system Prana, Subtle Fire (tejas) and Essence (ojas) are viewed as being pure expressions of the Five Elements within the physical body. These three subtle quintessential elements act upon the digestive and metabolic processes to produce seven substances that in turn create and maintain the body. The substances are Sap, Blood, Flesh, Fat, Bones, Marrow and Reproductive Tissue. These substances are produced in a progressive order, one substance being refined out of another. Furthermore the seven substances eventually serve to nourish the

Prana, Subtle Fire and Essence, which absorb rarefied aspects of the substances. Thus the substances and elements have a reciprocal relationship in maintaining homeostasis.

The Doshas for their part are thought to be grosser expressions of the three quintessential elements Prana, Subtle Fire and Essence. In healthy equilibrium the Doshas aid in the organizational integration of physiological processes, while a lack of equilibrium within the Doshas generates physiologic imbalance and eventually disease.

While Ayurveda and Chinese medicine both propose a Five Element model to organize the human physical terrain, in Ayurveda this model is simplified into a triune theory for understanding human physiology and energetic associations, the theory of the Three Doshas. This Ayurvedic model relates well to the Chinese medicine conceptualization of Yin, Yang and the potential Qi that arises from them, though the doshas cannot be equated with their Chinese counterparts. Kapha is related most closely to and exhibits the attributes of the Element Water and is thus analogous to Yin, while Pitta by relating to and displaying the qualities of the Fire Element corresponds to the image of Yang. Vata, which is primarily associated with the Air Element and is in charge of all forms of circulation, including that of Prana, is in accord with the Chinese idea of Qi.

In classical Ayurvedic physiology the three Doshas are further subdivided into five aspects each. While the five forms of Kapha manifest as special body lubricants and the five forms of Pitta appear as transformative substances, the five forms of Vata divide the body into spheres of influence, and this idea about Vata has a striking resemblance to the Chinese concept of the Triple Burner.

The Triple Burner has both systemic and local functions and orientations, and the three Burners correspond to the Forward-Moving (prana), Equalizing (samana) and Downward-Moving (apana) Vatas. The Forward-Moving (prana) Vata, situated between the throat and diaphragm, takes in and distributes the life force; this is similar to the function of the Cosmic and Ancestral Qi within the Upper Burner in Chinese medicine. The Equalizing (samana) Vata which is localized between the diaphragm and the navel and is in charge of digestion and assimilation is reminiscent of the Nutritive Qi that is centered within the Middle Burner. The Downward-Moving (apana) Vata, located in the lower trunk below the navel, has the function of pushing things downward and out of the body. In Chinese medicine Downward-Moving Vata corresponds to the location of the Lower Burner, although the descending function is specific to the Stomach's Organ Qi (see illustration 21).

As a whole unit the Triple Burner is perceived to arise out of the Original Qi, also known as the "moving Qi between the Kidneys" in the Lower Burner. The Original Qi, under the direction of the Triple Burner, is distributed throughout the body. The Triple Burner also distributes Protec-

AYURVEDIC   CHINESE MEDICINE

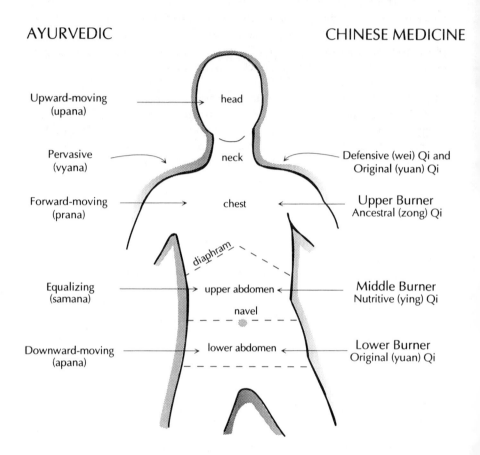

Upward-moving
(upana)   head

Pervasive   neck   Defensive (wei) Qi and
(vyana)   Original (yuan) Qi

Forward-moving   chest   Upper Burner
(prana)   Ancestral (zong) Qi

                              diaphram

Equalizing   upper abdomen   Middle Burner
(samana)   Nutritive (ying) Qi
                                    navel

Downward-moving   lower abdomen   Lower Burner
(apana)   Original (yuan) Qi

21. Vata's Five Forms and Triple Burner

tive Qi, which is directed upwards from the Lower Burner to the Lungs and then outward along the Meridians throughout the body's surface. The systemic function of the Triple Burner in distributing the Original and Protective Qi provides protection and nutrition and regulates the body's temperature. This global function of the Triple Burner is reminiscent of the function of Pervasive (vyana) Vata, for Pervasive Vata is said to emanate from the heart and to control the body's perspiration and temperature through its function of distributing blood and nutrients throughout the system. A fifth, Upward-Moving (udana) Vata, extends from the throat to the top of the head and appears to be the only component totally absent in the Chinese model. The following table summarizes the most important correspondences:

BURNER	QI TYPE	EFFECT	PRANA	ACTIVITY	LOCATION
UPPER	Ancestral	dispersion absorption	prana	forward	chest
MIDDLE	Nutritive	assimilation	samana	equalizing	upper abd.
LOWER	————	elimination storage	apana	downward	lower abd.
SYSTEMIC	Defensive Original	protection warmth	vyana	pervasive	upper

In Chinese medicine Blood is the counterpart of Qi, having a relationship to it which is analogous to the relationship of Yin to Yang; being more Yin, Blood tends to be injured easily by heat, a Yang force. In Ayurveda, disorders of blood are usually classified as Pitta disorders, since blood is most often injured by excessive heat. The concept of Blood is generally speaking a secondary feature of both systems, though as mentioned earlier, Sushruta and the Buddhists did advocate a system that included Blood as the fourth Dosha.

The Chinese developed a complex model to explain the functions of the various organs based on the energetic patterning of the individual organs in relationship with the body. These patterning images of the organs combine a broad range of ideas within the rubrics of traditional Chinese medical thought, including the Yin-Yang and the Five Element doctrines. According to the theory of the Meridians, the domain of an organ is not confined to its particular area in the body, but emanates its influence throughout the organism via its paired Meridian. Overall the Chinese placed great emphasis on the organs in terms of their energetics and in their role in pathology. Indian medicine's perspective of the organs, however, tended to be more practical in consequence perhaps of their more extensive anatomical knowledge. That is perhaps the reason why the organs perceived and described by classical Ayurveda resemble more closely with the descriptions of modern biomedical science. This is one reason Ayurveda seems easier to integrate with modern biomedicine than Chinese medicine (see illustration 22).

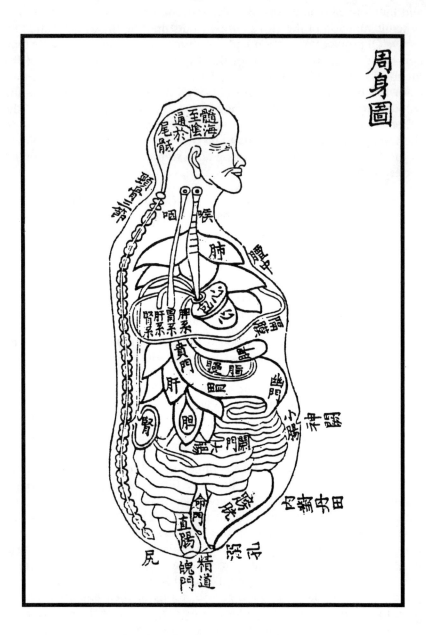

22. Classical Organ Drawing

A classical drawing, according to Chinese medicine, of the major organs (including their relative shape and position) along with the important anatomical landmarks of the head and trunk.

Despite differences in their treatment of the organs, similarities also abound. For example, the Ayurvedic doctrine of the preeminent role of the lungs and large intestine in the absorption of Prana helps to explain the pairing of these two organs in the Chinese system. Chinese medicine's explanation of why the Lungs and Large Intestine are connected is based on structural manifestation. The cool "white" Organs Lungs and Large Intestine are outside of and so surround, buffer and restrain the inside, hot, "red" Organs Heart and Small Intestine respectively. The lungs and heart manifest together a rhythmic motion, as do the intestines in the form of their peristaltic rhythm. This outside-inside structural relationship compliments and contrasts their energetic relationship within the Five Elements, which states that the Fire (Heart and Small Intestine) controls Metal (Lung and Large Intestine). These two Organ pairs are the only coupled Elemental Organs that are physically separated, by the diaphragm; all the other pairs are coupled because of their proximity and their similar physiological processes.

Ayurveda proposes an energetic connection between Lung and Large Intestine that is not clearly made in Chinese medicine. In Ayurveda the lungs perform "immediate" absorption of Prana into the body from ingested air, while the large intestine performs "delayed" absorption by extracting Prana from ingested food. Although Chinese medicine also accepts the Lungs to take in Cosmic Qi, it does not mention any significant absorption of Qi by the Large Intestine.

Chinese medicine and Ayurveda both affirm that the emotions have specific sites of resonance within the body, sites which correspond to various organs. In general, both systems assign the same imbalanced effects from the same emotions; anger, for example, is said by both to relate to the liver and gallbladder. This practical understanding offers a unique and clinically valuable tool to trace the psycho-physiologic manifestations of illness. From the Chinese perspective, specific imbalanced emotions generate directional changes in the flow of Qi, thus deranging it. Imbalanced emotions also negatively influence the organs and/or related structures according to their Five-Element resonance. In Ayurveda imbalanced emotions will disturb the corresponding Dosha, but the manifestation of the imbalance may appear in any part of the body, depending on a variety of other factors.

3

Consciousness

The word "consciousness" is often taken in English to include all conscious, subconscious and unconscious faculties of awareness. Neither Sanskrit nor Chinese offers an equivalent all-embracing synonym for the English word. Nor is it easy to compare the many distinctive terms in ancient India and China to elucidate their unique ideas on the subject of consciousness, for their concepts tend to diverge.

Though Ayurveda makes selective use of many Indian schools of thought on the subject, including the Nyaya-Vaisheshika and the Mimamsa, it is mainly indebted to the Sankhya philosophy for its ideas on consciousness. Indian culture, science and religion seem always to have been preoccupied with understanding and explaining consciousness, a preoccupation which produced the rich body of knowledge that includes the science of Ayurveda.

The Chinese approach to this question, on the other hand, is rather physical, more archaic and down to earth. Chinese philosophy and religion view the physical body and Spirit as a continuum of each other, expressing the dynamic dualism that permeates nature according to the Yin-Yang theory. Chinese medicine never significantly added to or developed new theories of consciousness beyond these ancient cultural ideas in spite of the later influence of Indian Buddhism.

In the Chinese classics the Spirit (shen) is considered to encompass and regulate all aspects of consciousness; mind, cognition, intellect, ego functioning and so on. Spirit, being an integrative force, is centered in the Heart, though it utilizes the physical brain for functional purposes. Furthermore, according to the Chinese doctrine of the Five Elements, the four other Yin Organs assist the Spirit housed in the Heart in storing subtle aspects of consciousness. The most important of these psycho-physical forces are the Spiritual Soul (hun) housed in the Liver and the Animal Soul (po) housed in the Lungs (there were actually said to be three Spiritual souls and seven Animal souls). These two soul groups form a polarity, functioning to primarily generate a person's unique temperament; and secondarily to govern the fate of the individual after death. The Kidneys are said to house the Will, while the Spleen for its part is believed to house the Intellect.

By contrast the Indian classics distinguish between a causal body, a subtle body (consisting of mind, intellect and senses) and a physical body, all connected together by an organizing principle (ego or ahamkara). The soul (purusa) which is of a pure transcendental nature, being self- luminous and eternally conscious, is set apart from all three of these bodies. Embodied consciousness operates in accord with the cosmic tendencies of the Three Attributes (gunas; i.e. sattva, rajas and tamas), the intellect providing the physical basis for cognitive and discriminatory abilities while the ego provides self-awareness and individuation to the personality. The mind motivates, supervises and receives the impressions of the sense organs that are constituted from the Five Elements that form the gross body. The mind thinks, measures, and makes decisions. Ayurveda describes the seat of this mind-intellect-ego complex as the 'heart'; under certain conditions this 'heart' is actually the brain, while in others it is the physical heart in the chest. At any particular moment, whatever organ consciousness concentrates in is considered the 'heart' at that time.

4
Disease Causation

oth Indian and Chinese cultures recognized the fact that living in
harmony with nature and human society is a prerequisite for perfect
health. Disorientation or interruption of this organic relationship with the
physical, social or spiritual environment is seen in both Ayurveda and Chinese medicine as the primary cause of ill health. Both traditions agree that
every human being has an inherently unique physical and psychological
profile that arises from predisposed hereditary and karmic factors and develops according to the conditioning received from one's social milieu.
Each individual by virtue of his or her constitution will react differently to
environmental conditions and psychological stresses, and the complexion
of this reaction will determine whether or not one is able to live in harmony with nature. In Ayurveda people are differentiated according to the
Three Doshas while in Chinese medicine the theories of Yin-Yang and the
Five Elements provide the basis for understanding a person's constitution
and susceptibility to illness.

Indian and Chinese medicine both concur that disease can arise
either within the body or from the exterior environment, depending on
constitutional precipitating factors. Chinese medicine considers interior
disorders to arise, primarily, from disturbance within the seven emotions
and, secondarily, from the organs. Ayurveda views the "allurement" of the
mind by sense objects and its "willfulness" in gratifying these desires as
the fundamental cause of all disease, since improper gratification will disturb the digestive fire.

In general, contemporary Chinese medicine tends to put its greatest emphasis on the external climatic and endogenous organ causes for
disease, while Ayurveda places its greatest emphasis on the role of digestion in the generation of disease. Almost all diseases in Ayurveda are said
to be traceable to weakness of the digestive fire. In Chinese physiology, the
internal fire that warms the body, regulates temperature and kindles digestion is referred to as Yang Qi. Unlike Ayurveda, internal fire in Chinese
medicine does not assume this central role in disease causation.

External causative factors are spoken about as forces in nature that
injure the body, and both systems use remarkably similar ideas and terms
to describe this form of etiology. For example the climatic factors of cold
and damp are known to aggravate the Kapha Dosha in Ayurveda, while in

Chinese medicine these external forces are said to increase the Yin within the body. The chart below lists some of the correspondences that exist between external etiologic factors:

AYURVEDA		CHINESE MEDICINE	
DOSHA	CLIMATIC FACTOR	SUBSTANCE	CLIMATIC FACTOR
Vata	wind & cold-dryness	Qi	wind & dryness
Pitta	heat & humidity	Yang	heat & summer heat
Kapha	cold-dampness	Yin	cold & dampness

Wind and dryness according to Chinese medicine are classically associated with the Yang. In the chart above these two climatic factors are associated with the Qi because wind and dryness affect the Liver and Lungs respectively. These organs are paramount in the circulation of Qi throughout the body, and clinical observation shows that these climatic factors do in fact disturb the circulation of Qi.

Indian and Chinese medicine also agree that the transitions or junctions of the seasons are crucial times during which illness may arise if the body's resistance to disease and adaptability to the environment is low. For example, Kapha predominates during childhood and Pitta during adulthood. Puberty and adolescence form the transition between these two "seasons" of life, and teenagers accordingly are prone to developing physical and mental imbalances. Menopause and its male equivalent, form the junction between the Pitta-predominant adult years and the Vata-dominated later years.

Both systems also emphasize the need to understand the effects of daily cycles on the human body. The Chinese perceive night and day as expressions of Yin and Yang, and label diurnal and nocturnal flows of energy through the Meridians and organs. In the Ayurveda paradigm, Pitta predominates during midday and midnight, Kapha in early morning and early evening, and Vata at the two junctions (dawn and dusk), but there is also a relative overall predominance of Pitta during the day and Kapha during the night. Likewise while the Indian year is sub-divided into six seasons according to the effects of annual time on the Doshas, it is also divided into two halves according to whether the sun is "withdrawing" energy from the earth (as it does when we are closest to it, during the summer) or "releasing" energy to the earth (during the winter). Similarly the Chinese ascribed each season to an Element which reflected its innate nature whose forces could enhance or disrupt the body's equilibrium depending on the circumstance.

All diseases create either a deficiency or an excess condition. In Ayurveda both conditions eventually weaken the physical or mental digestive fire, and give rise to the production of Digestive Toxins, a pathological autotoxin composed of partially digested material that clogs the system and engenders unique symptoms. Digestive Toxins in their turn aggravate Vata's circulatory functions, and Vata then further aggravates Pitta and Kapha. Eventually the imbalanced Doshas spread throughout the body, dispersing disease farther afield.

Chinese medical thought has a similar concept of pathological autotoxins in the form of Phlegm and, to a lesser extent, Stagnant Blood. According to this theory Phlegm originates from a disturbance of water metabolism in the body, mostly but not exclusively from the digestive system. Stagnant Blood is the result of trauma or injury wherein blood pools and coagulates in a particular location. Both of these result in the disruption of normal circulation, complication of disease, and the manifestation of unusual symptoms. They are considered extra factors, neither purely internal nor external.

In a broader sense Chinese medicine believes that most diseases originate as an excess condition which will eventually transform itself into a deficiency state in chronic illness. The more Organs and Elements the disease pattern is dispersed in, the greater its severity. In Ayurveda the Doshas are believed to generate states of either excess or deficiency, though most common patterns are conditions of excess. And the greater number of Doshas, Tissues, Wastes and Pathways that get involved in an illness, obviously the greater its severity. Additionally, Ayurveda maintains that any disorder that matches the constitutional pattern of the patient is more difficult to cure than a disorder which is different in nature from the constitutional type.

Whereas Ayurveda describes a certain sequence of pathways for a particular disease to penetrate within, Chinese medicine ascribes the main role for the spread of disease to the Meridian network. For example, an external climatic factor, such as wind, will enter the body through the skin and respiratory tract first, and then move progressively inward to the organs via the Meridians. And in case of internal disorders the Meridians convey the signs and symptoms of the disease to the periphery.

Ayurveda generally tends to be comparatively linear in its conceptualization of disease progression, while the Chinese propound a somewhat circular sequential order in this context. Both systems believe that healing once begun often causes the disease to retrace its path in the opposite direction to exit out of the body.

5
Diagnosis

Ayurveda and Chinese Medicine utilize fairly similar diagnostic methods based on sensory observation and questioning by the practitioner. In both systems this process is a synthetic one that allows the practitioner a great deal of latitude in choosing from an assortment of investigatory procedures. Examination of the pulse is still the preeminent diagnostic technique within both traditions, and the methodology employed in the two systems differs only slightly. Moreover the interpretations given to pulse analysis in both show a wide concordance. The general characteristics of the three Doshas and their analogous Chinese counterpart pulses are: Vata or Qi-floating, empty and irregular; Pitta or Yang-tight, rapid and wiry or full; and Kapha or Yin- large, slow and deep.

Both systems postulate that the pulses reflect both the overall level of vitality and the diseased condition of the individual. One major difference between the two in pulse diagnosis, however, is that the Chinese utilize the pulse to determine the conditions of the individual organs and their associated Meridians as also to the pernicious influences and state of the substances; whereas in Ayurveda, the state of the Doshas by pulse diagnosis is of paramount concern, reflecting the lack of emphasis on organs as mentioned earlier. The state of the body's Qi or Prana, too, is emulated in the pulse, and therefore pulse examination is used to prognosticate the immanence of death as well.

Because Ayurveda acquired the procedure of pulse examination later in its development, Ayurvedic doctors originally relied on such observations as facial color, tongue, eyes, gait, etc.; questioning, and inference for their diagnoses. Urinalysis, commonly used in India today, also seems to have been acquired later from the Tibetans (see illustration 23).

A great deal of similarity exists in the methodology for observation of the tongue for diagnostic purposes. In each system the tongue is divided into thirds—the tip, middle portion and root—which are linked, respectively, to the chest, upper and lower abdomen, and the organs therein. Observations pertaining to the tongue's color, shape, texture and coating are analyzed in both traditions, primarily, for the presence of heat or cold, and secondarily for other pathogenic factors.

In Ayurveda a practitioner learns the art of prognosis, which incorporates a highly intuitive and spiritual understanding of life. This deep

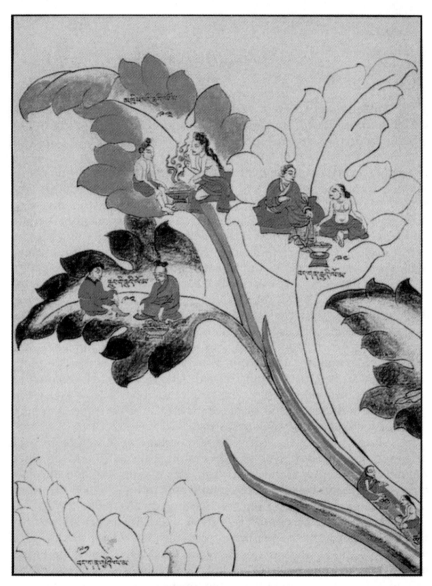

23. Tibetan Urinalysis

Urinalysis, which entails visual observation of the urine for diagnosis, originated in Tibetan medicine. This drawing illustrates that the urine is differentiated according to the aggravated dosha. Thus the three leaves on this branch show from *lower left clockwise to the right*: Vata urine, Pitta urine, and Kapha urine.

study reflects on the doctors' skills and hence reputation as much as does diagnosis and resultant treatment. The prognosis is determined through a variety of procedures: a thorough examination to determine the general constitution of the patient, the nature and stage of the illness, and a consideration of a myriad of omens including the patient's dreams.

Chinese medicine is largely devoid of the systematic spiritual aspect of this type of prognosis as a result of the abandonment of spiritual beliefs within its philosophical rationale. Thus one finds a greater belief in spirit possession, effects of curses, and other occult influences in Ayurveda than in modern Chinese medicine.

Following diagnostic inquiry, the physician must organize and differentiate the information elicited by the procedures. While Ayurveda tries to utilize the Dosha theory as exclusively as possible in its pathology, with the addition of allied concepts such as Digestive Toxins; Chinese medicine employs a wider variety of patterning frameworks. The most commonly used theories referred to are the Eight Guiding Principles based on the Yin-Yang doctrine, the Five Element model, and patterns based on the Organ theory and Climatic influences. Both medical systems delineate the signs and symptoms of common diseases that have specific identifiable patterns, such as anxiety, jaundice, seizures, and indigestion.

Permutations of patterns are however common to both. Just as in the Dosha theory of Ayurveda, derangements of two or even three Doshas can simultaneously exist, Chinese medicine also recognizes the presence of multiple patterns in most patients. And through an analysis of each patterning model the complex clinical presentations of each patient are more easily understood. Theoretically Chinese medicine with its inherent diversity of models is less constrained than Ayurveda, wherein the Dosha model predominates, for in Chinese medicine if a practitioner is ineffective with a treatment based on the strategy of a particular disease model, the condition may be reexamined and treated utilizing an approach outlined by a different patterning model. In practice, however, Ayurvedic physicians do usually evince the ability to successfully manipulate the Dosha theory when a revaluation of therapy is called for.

6
Treatment

*T*he purpose of therapy in Ayurveda and Chinese medicine is to a achieve balance within the body and mind. In Ayurveda a person's lifestyle, diet, psychological make-up and spiritual beliefs are actively addressed in formulating an overall strategy, while contemporary Chinese medicine focuses more on addressing a patient's specific problems or disease. Ayurveda as a body of practice emphasizes treating a person's constitution to a far greater extent than does Chinese Medicine. Viewed this way, these two systems can be perceived as complementary to each other: Ayurveda tends to have a more long-term perspective, while Chinese medicine focuses primarily on immediate relief of symptoms and disease.

In Chinese medicine the broad treatment strategy for any sort of disease pattern is to sedate Excess patterns first and tonify Deficient patterns thereafter. Similarly according to Ayurveda, conditions of excess involving derangement of the Doshas and/or accumulation of toxins should first be redressed before rejuvenative techniques (rasayana) are to be employed to tonify and build up the system. Common forms of therapy used by both these traditions are: massage and manipulation; bonesetting; surgery; various methods of cautery; dietary regimentation; for internal usage medicines prepared from plants, mineral and animal products; and exercise.

Chinese medicine's unique field of expertise has been acupuncture, which for some obscure reason was never transmitted into India until this century. Acupuncture has been openly embraced and popularized by many nations during the last twenty years, and its powerful treatment potential and utilization for pain control was instrumental in generating much scientific and public interest in not only acupuncture itself, but also in all of Asian medicine. Ayurveda's unique modality is in its Purification therapy (panchakarma), which is a complete system for detoxifying the body and initiating balance unto the system.

Both systems base most of their prescriptions on plant-derived substances, though due to the enduring influence of the ancient alchemical arts, Ayurveda utilizes mineral preparations to a greater extent than does Chinese medicine, but Chinese medicine's pharmacopeia is replete with many more animal parts than does that of Ayurveda. Both systems have sophisticated methods of preparing their remedies, particularly those which include toxic plants and minerals which need to be detoxified by elaborate processes. The medicinal preparations appear in a wide variety of forms as detailed earlier.

Both Ayurveda and Chinese medicine have, through their understanding of the unique properties of plants, minerals and animal substances, achieved a sophisticated knowledge of how substances interact. Each system thereby developed myriads of synergistic compounds whose total effect surpasses the sum of its individual ingredients, and in each country this accumulated knowledge was recorded in texts which specialized in materia medica and formulation. This continuity of knowledge has allowed practitioners of both healing arts access to centuries of data collected on the benefits, limitations, interactions and possible side-effects of substances. Even today hundreds of the medicinal formulas used in China and India both, are based upon ancient prescriptions, some of them over 2,000 years old!

Chinese medicine classifies the medicinal substances used in prescriptions by their taste, temperature, direction of action and effect upon Meridians and Organs; whereas Ayurveda's categorization pertains to taste, potency, post-digestive effect and special power. Ayurveda distinguishes six different tastes—sweet, sour, salty, pungent, bitter and astringent—of which only astringent is not found in Chinese medicine's five classes of tastes. In Chinese medicine rather, two separate tastes, astringent and aromatic, are used to denote, respectively, a substance's ability to prevent edema and to awaken the digestive fire and spirit. Even in Ayurveda astringent is regarded by some authorities to be an action instead of a taste, since astringent causes tissues to contract, which is why it makes the mouth pucker. According to Chinese medicine each taste has a distinct effect upon the Qi, a concept useful in understanding the action of a substance in totality.

In both Chinese medicine and Ayurveda the tastes are linked to each system's version of the Five Elements. While Chinese medicine associates only one element with a particular taste, Ayurveda associates two elements with each taste. The concepts of taste in the two systems are however in general agreement with regard to their effects on the physical body, though there is a divergence of opinion in the case of salty taste: salt is considered by Ayurveda to be heating, while Chinese medicine regards it to be cooling.

In Chinese medicine, salt's cooling nature is congruent with its close association to the water element. Salt has a Yin, softening quality that is in harmony with the innate nature of water. Indeed, ocean water and human blood contain the same relative proportion of salt. Internally, salt regulates body fluid levels, primarily through its effect upon the kidneys. It softens and disperses congealed Qi, loosens the muscles, and cools the blood. Goiter is an example of a condition that arises from internal heat and Qi stagnation, and may be influenced by salt. Chinese medicine utilizes salt or salty herbs to cool and soften the tissues, and in higher amounts salt purges the intestines, thereby reducing internal body heat.

Ayurveda views salt as heating because it creates a burning sensation when placed in the mouth or upon an open wound, stimulates digestive fire, promotes retention of body fluids, and inhibits perspiration, resulting in increased internal heat. But Ayurveda does recognize salt's softening effect. Perhaps these varied views on salt's cooling and heating ability reflect, respectively, its initial or prolonged effects on the body.

Classification of substances by tendency to cause heating or cooling is called a substance's temperature in Chinese medicine and its potency in Ayurveda. Ayurveda's concept of potency actually embraces other polarities of a substance's action including heavy and light, and wet and dry, thus conforming to the Yin-Yang theory and to the Chinese concept of direction of action. Unique to Chinese formulation is the concept of a substance's effect on particular energetic Meridians and Organs, while the idea of a substance's post-digestive and special effect is distinctly specific to Ayurveda. For comparative purposes, a brief outline of twelve medicinal substances utilized by both Chinese and Indian medicine has been provided in Appendix I.

As regards to the process of drug administration, Ayurveda employs a greater variety of preparations and methods of delivery. Ayurvedic formulations include expressed plant juices; powders and pastes; hot and cold decoctions; pills; wines; medicated fats, oils and butters; and mineral and gemstone preparations. In Ayurveda, subject to the nature of the illness, medicines may be administered orally, through the nostrils, via the anus (in the form of an enema), dropped into the ear, or applied over the skin. In contrast, Chinese medicine relies, almost exclusively, on the oral administration of decoctions, wines and pills; only for external injuries are liniments and plasters applied topically.

7
Primal Distinctions

Given their many similarities, it is instructive to examine some of the reasons for the differences which exist between these two quite similar medical systems. Variance of climate is certainly one reason for differences in theory. China is situated generally further to the north of India and has mostly a cooler, temperate climate, and therefore the medical preoccupation has always been to keep the body warm. This concern may perhaps also be deduced from the impetus for concepts such as the Triple Burner. India's climate, however, being more tropical, Ayurveda has necessarily been more concerned with keeping the body cool yet maintaining a strong digestive fire.

It is also evident though, that there are profound differences in Indian and Chinese thought patterns. The civilization of India that developed Ayurveda has a tendency to promote linear thinking, as reflected in the linear script it developed for its languages. Chinese thought, on the other hand, is markedly more circular and pattern-oriented, as evinced by China's refusal to renounce its symbolic language based on pictographic characters. Since most human knowledge is couched in language, the structure of the language in which a theory is expressed inevitably helps to determine its orientation.

Political differences have also played a part in the development of these medical systems. China during its long history, has enjoyed several periods of unification which promoted social homogeneity, and its relatively more stable social setting may have encouraged medical innovation, providing Chinese medicine with a range of theoretical models and practices that are inherently more diverse than Ayurveda's. India has never been as homogenized as China, even though all the foreign conquerors who arrived and set up house eventually became assimilated as a new sub-group within India's diverse cultural mosaic, at least until the coming of the Europeans. Perpetual political turmoil may well have played a role in the codification and standardization of Ayurveda during its long history, for it flourished for centuries despite frequent changes in government. That the British attempted to "outlaw" Ayurveda was consistent with their adamant refusal to "go native," a refusal which probably facilitated their successful political unification of the subcontinent.

The extreme complexity of both of these ancient civilizations makes any sort of facile conclusions hazardous. It seems, however, likely that as exposure of traditions to each other increases, the awareness of the ways in which and the extent to which cultural traits have affected medical concepts will gradually become more apparent. Hopefully it will then become easier to get rid off many of the prevalent cultural biases from the systems, facilitating their communion, if not integration.

8
Integrating Traditions

Since Ayurveda in general, focuses more on understanding and treating constitutional types, whereas Chinese medicine predominantly addresses specific disease patterns, these two approaches towards healthy living are potentially complementary. For example, from a Chinese medical perspective Kapha displays the general characteristics of hypo-activity. This manifests in the body as a tendency towards heaviness and coldness due to deficiency of Yang (i.e. heat). Body fluids easily accumulate due to impaired circulation, and a diminution of digestive and metabolic functioning takes place. The diseases of dampness, cold and phlegm fall within the domain of Kapha. The mental disposition eminently distinct for Kapha is a dullness of mind that causes possessiveness, melancholy, calmness, and a tendency to over-indulgence. In Chinese medicine these are primarily the syndromes associated with the Spleen and Stomach, and secondarily with those involving the Lungs, Kidneys and Bladder, that appear to be most closely related with Kapha. Both Chinese medicine and Ayurveda agree that Pungent taste, keeping warm, dispersing and drying conditions, all Yang in nature, are ideal for countering excess of Kapha.

Pitta displays the general characteristic of hyperactivity, a decidedly Yang attribute. In the body this manifests as lightness and heat due to deficiency in the body's Yin. This condition of excess heat injures the Blood, and increases the digestive and metabolic activity. In Chinese medicine heat disorders (fire and summerheat), including the pattern of heat in the Blood, are found to correspond with Pitta. The mental disposition of this Dosha involves sharpness of mind, acute discrimination, aggressive disposition, anger and jealousness. In Chinese medicine the patterns of the Liver and Gallbladder, and secondarily those of the Heart, Small Intestine and Kidneys, relate most closely with Pitta. Foods and medicines that posses the bitter taste are best to sedate Pitta, followed by sweet and astringent. There is consensus between Ayurveda and Chinese medicine that Bitter, due to its inherent cooling, clearing and drying properties, and its Yin nature, best neutralizes Pitta.

Vata has the general characteristic of being mobile and unstable like the wind and generates a sense of constant shifting in body and mind. In excess this manifests as pains and sensations that are not fixed in location or duration, and in a tendency towards dryness. Vata is closely associated with Prana in Ayurveda; and the latter in Chinese medicine can be likened to Qi disorders. Thus Vata's manifestation will correspond to deficiency states of Qi and derangement of its circulation. The mental state of Vata reveals a changeable mental disposition marked by fear, moodiness, nervousness, anxiety and restlessness. In Chinese medicine Vata imbalance primarily correlates with the Organ patterns related to the Liver and Lung, and secondarily with Heart Protector, Triple Burner, and Large Intestine syndromes. Salty foods and medicines are best suited to stabilize Vata, but to a lesser degree sour and sweet foods and medicines are also effective. Though Ayurveda and Chinese medicine disagree on the salty taste's effects, both systems do agree that salt does possess a softening capability.

Historically, the greatest cross-fertilization between Indian and Chinese systems has occurred in the field of the therapeutic uses of plant, mineral and animal products; and hence there already exists a certain commonality of practice in Internal Medicine which may turn out to have a potential for efficacy enhancement. For example, Ayurveda could profitably absorb Chinese medicine's methods of formulation and its understanding of the Tastes according to their effect upon the Qi; whereas Chinese medicine could integrate the Ayurvedic concepts of Post-Digestive effect and the principle of the ten Pairs of Qualities to its advantage.

Massage, bloodletting and moxibustion are common adjunctive practices of Chinese medicine. While bloodletting is indicated in heat disorders and moxibustion in cold patterns, massage while useful in many types of illnesses is most effective in disorders of Qi circulation. These modalities are used similarly in Ayurveda. Below is a breakdown of these three adjunctive techniques, as well as other beneficial practices, according to the Dosha alleviated:

VATA	PITTA	KAPHA
massage	bloodletting	moxibustion
sweating	cold water therapy	heat treatments
plentiful sleep	tranquil environment	vigorous exercise
avoiding wind & cold	cool environment	sunbathing
avoiding overwork	relaxation	stimulation

In the authors' experience, acupuncture is useful in most types of patterns and should benefit any Dosha constitution. However, by modification of the acupuncture technique in accordance with the patient's main Dosha imbalance, the efficacy of acupuncture can be greatly enhanced. The following chart gives general parameters of acupuncture treatment according to the three Dosha types:

DOSHA	INTENSITY OF STIMULATION	NUMBER OF NEEDLES	LENGTH OF NEEDLING TIME	DEPTH OF INSERTION
VATA	mild	few	short	superficial
PITTA	moderate	moderate	medium	medial
KAPHA	strong	many	long	deep

From an Ayurvedic perspective, the general role of acupuncture is in balancing Prana and harmonizing the relationship between the physical and mental body, since the Prana operates between these two bodies. Certainly acupuncture is one modality that would be of great benefit to incorporate within Ayurveda, though it may be difficult to harmonize the conceptual model of the Meridian Network and Organ Images with Ayurvedic theory without adopting the Chinese Yin-Yang and Five Element perspective.

The Purification practices in Ayurveda similarly can be of great utility when incorporated into the treatment strategy of Chinese medicine. The purification of the body accelerates the healing of the patient as well as enhances the effectiveness of any therapies that follow, such as acupuncture, exercise or Internal Medicine. Yet purification can only be initiated when the patient's symptoms become mild and non-threatening. Therefore, acupuncture can be used prior to Purification therapy to curtail the symptoms.

In any event, clinical experimentation is likely to be the key to any possible eventual détente between these two titans, for theoretical integration of two systems which follow separate modes of thought and divergent doctrines is much more problematical. Since these divergent outlooks are complementary, however, some sort of correlation between them does seem worthy of serious study.

CONCLUSION

*A*yurveda and Chinese medicine are both living systems of medicine with ancient roots, the oldest continuously practiced and recorded medical traditions in the world. Both systems are based on a natural empiricism coupled with intuition that was practiced by the doctor-sages of old. The study of their history shows many points of contact and many attempts (some successful, others not) to cross-fertilize ideas and practices, the early Buddhists having been particularly instrumental in facilitating this contact and exchange.

Fundamental to both systems is the belief that an individual who lives in accord with the laws of Nature remains healthy, and that deviation from Nature's path is the root cause of all ill health and suffering. Chinese medicine uses the concepts of the Tao, Yin and Yang and the Five Elements to explain the working of Nature, while Ayurveda bases itself on the Sankhya philosophy and uses the theory of Doshas, Five Elements and the Three Attributes (equilibrium, activity and inertia) to explain its vision of the natural order. Although Chinese and Indian doctrines do share certain common themes, they are essentially unique, and their concepts cannot be interchanged in their entirety.

One common feature of both medical paradigms is the belief in an essential life force, called Prana by the Indians and Qi by the Chinese. Both paradigms have remarkably similar ideas on the nature, transportation, origin and importance of this substance, and they are in general agreement in their views of the other substances of life such as blood and essence. Mind and body are understood as inseparable by both systems, though their explanations about the structure of consciousness do diverge.

Etiological understanding is linked to each system's explanation of the forces of Nature, and images of these external forces are used to explain how deviation from the laws of Nature manifests as symptoms of disease in the body. Both systems use the natural sensory skills of the physician to interpret the patient's symptoms, with striking similarities in diagnostic techniques, particularly in palpation of the pulse, visual inspection, listening and questioning.

The current worldwide explosion of interest in botanical medicine and acupuncture has increased the profile of and generated enthusiasm for research into both of these Asian systems of medicine. We believe that botanical medicine and the practice of acupuncture are probably the key areas in which the relationship between these two systems can be immediately strengthened. Plant, minerals and even certain prescriptions are known to have been incorporated into each others' pharmacopeias; and the similarity and practicality of their use of a substance's taste and temperature in its classification is a topic that is being widely studied today in modern botanical medicine.

Although integration on several levels seems directly possible, much experimental work will be needed to make it more widely applicable. Perhaps one feasible way to initiate this process may start with introduction of inter-disciplinary courses into the curricula of both Ayurvedic and Chinese Medical colleges. Synergizing the overall characteristics of both disciplines can ultimately lead to the development of a truly holistic science of energetic medicine in the future.

APPENDIX I

Comparison of Some Important Medicinal Substances

China and India have traded and exchanged much information on the use of plants, minerals and animal products for food and medicinal purposes over their long history. The merchants, priests and scholars who over the past two millennia sought new sources of medicines undoubtedly exchanged information about each culture's use of drugs. About a quarter of the plants listed in the Chinese classic *Compendium of Materia Medica* (*Ben Cao Gang Mu*), which was written in 1590 A.D. by Li Shi Zhen and was considered the most extensive materia medica in its time, are common to both India and China. Many of the plants listed in this Chinese materia medica were in fact imported from India. Trade and information historically also went the other way, over the Himalayas to influence Ayurveda's formulations, and new medicinal substances are still being introduced into the market place in both India and China. Ginseng root, for example, is now being cultivated and sold in India.

In this appendix a representative group of twelve substances which are common to both traditions, ten of plant origin and one each from the mineral and animal kingdoms, is discussed from both perspectives. About half the drugs mentioned below are native to both countries, and the rest were originally trade commodities native to one or the other. This comparative survey includes a brief historical background, each drug's Latin, Sanskrit and Chinese names, and the part(s) of the source plant, mineral or animal which was traditionally used.

As will become evident hereafter, the Chinese and Ayurvedic systems categorized and utilized most medicinal substances in approximately similar ways. The general uniformity of opinion on the taste and temperature properties of the substances among both systems is perhaps due to the fact that both taste and temperature are deduced directly through sensory feedback and physical interaction with the substance. Those divergences of opinion which do occur may be partially explained by the subtle changes a plant goes through in adapting to a different habitat, and partially by the specific uses that each discipline emphasizes in accordance with its own medical paradigm. Also, the context of the whole materia medica affects how a substance may be emphasized, so that what is a minor remedy in one system may in the other be portrayed as an indispensable drug.

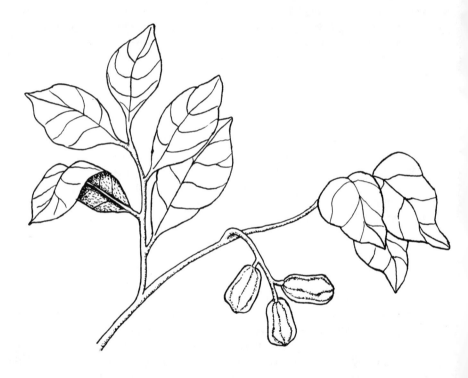

24. Chebulic Myrobalan, *Terminalia chebula*

CHEBULIC MYROBALAN   BOTANICAL NAME: *Terminalia chebula*
CHINESE NAME: he zi   SANSKRIT NAME: haritaki
PART USED: fruit
TASTE: bitter, astringent & sour (c) / all tastes except salty,
with astringent predominating (a)
TEMPERATURE: neutral (c) / heating (a)

Chebulic myrobalan holds a position of high esteem in Ayurveda, perhaps its most important plant. Chebulic myrobalan's Sanskrit name (haritaki) has the triple meaning of taking away all diseases (harayet), of being green in natural color (harita) and of growing in the abode of Lord Shiva (Hara), the Himalayas (considered the plant's ideal habitat). Since Charaka's time chebulic myrobalan fruit has been considered a powerful tonic and rejuvenative that "never causes harm to a person who takes it." Chebulic myrobalan found favor wherever it went, in Greco-Roman, Tibetan, Chinese and Arabic medicine, being praised by Avicenna, the great 11th century Muslim physician, and extolled in the *Four Tantras* (*Gyushi*), Tibet's preeminent medical text, as the "king of medicines." So sacred is chebulic myrobalan to Tibetans that it is the Medicine Buddha is visualized holding in his extended right hand in a gesture of giving. Tibetan medicine utilizes every part of this plant for medicinal purposes.

Ayurveda utilizes not one but three myrobalans, however; the other two being Emblica officinalis (amalaki) and Terminalia belerica (bibhitaki). The three together form triphala ("three fruits"), a remedy par excellence for regulating and toning the digestive tract, and one of Ayurveda's foremost prescriptions. Ayurveda considers chebulic myrobalan calming to all Doshas, and especially beneficial for reducing Vata, for though the fruit is predominantly astringent in taste it is warming in its inherent attribute and its post-digestive effect is sweet. Chebulic myrobalan's main therapeutic function is to scrape away digestive toxins from the digestive tract and the tissues (especially the blood). It is much used in abdominal distension, malabsorption, jaundice, tumors, urinary infections, edema, and in both constipation and diarrhea. Chebulic myrobalan is said to rejuvenate both the body (especially the colon and lungs) and mind, to impart wisdom and intelligence, and to increase longevity. This makes it ideal for use in chronic conditions such as asthma (in which case its jam is consumed or its coarse powder is smoked), prolapses of various organs, abnormal discharges (spermatorrhea, leucorrhea, and sweating), and bleeding gums.

Chebulic myrobalan was first mentioned in Chinese medicine in the *Materia Medica of Medicinal Properties* (*Yao Xing Ben Cao*), a text published around 600 A.D., as a fruit originating from India. Nowadays it is grown in the southern Chinese provinces of Yunnan, Guangdong and Guangxi. Chebulic myrobalan has no special status in Chinese medicine. It is said to bind up the intestines, and to be useful in treating dysentery and chronic diarrhea due to either internal heat or coldness (which is why Chinese medicine considers it to have a neutral temperature). Also, since chebulic myrobalan is said to contain the lung's Qi it is able to stop coughing, relieve asthma, and soothe the throat. Chinese medicine administers the fruit in the roasted form for intestinal symptoms, and in the raw form for respiratory complaints.

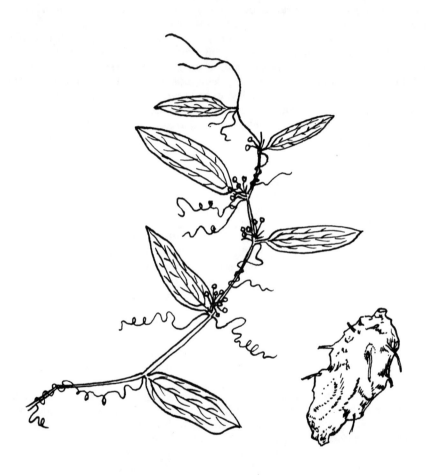

25. China Root, *Smilax glabra, Smilax chinensis*

CHINA ROOT   BOTANICAL NAME: *Smilax glabra, Smilax chinensis*
CHINESE NAME: tu fu ling   SANSKRIT NAME: dwipautra
PART USED: root   TASTE: bitter & sweet
TEMPERATURE: neutral (c) / slightly cooling; although some authorities
say mildly heating (a)

Of the many varieties of smilax or sarsaparilla throughout Asia, one highly regarded species called china root was exported to India under the name "chob-chini." This became an important Chinese trade commodity with the spread of syphilis from the New World, after the 15th century. According to Chinese medicine, china root's main use is in treating syphilis and chronic skin disorders (ulcers, gout and hot boils) which are characterized by the presence of damp-heat. In fact the increased importance of smilax in Chinese medicine occurred in response to the spread of syphilis. Furthermore, china root eliminates systemic damp-heat which may display itself as rheumatic joint pain, difficult, cloudy and painful urination, or jaundice.

Ayurvedic medicine utilizes china root (and the other species of sarsaparilla) as deep-acting blood cleansers for more or less the same physical complaints as does Chinese medicine. One major difference is that Ayurveda ascribes to china root a purifying and tranquilizing effect upon the mind, which makes it useful in treating disorders of the nervous system such as epilepsy and insanity. Generally, sarsaparilla reduces Vata and purifies Pitta (and so improves Essential Fire), while being neutral in effect on Kapha. It has a slight tonic effect upon the reproductive organs and is used externally to treat venereal sores and herpes.

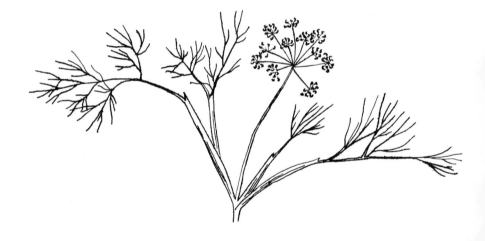

26. Fennel, *Foeniculum vulgare*

FENNEL   BOTANICAL NAME: *Foeniculum vulgare*
CHINESE NAME: xiao hui xiang   SANSKRIT NAME: shatapuspa
PART USED: seeds   TASTE: pungent (c) / sweet & pungent (a)
TEMPERATURE: slightly warm

Fennel is thought to have originally come from the Mediterranean area, and to have slowly spread eastward over the centuries. The first mention of fennel in the Chinese texts is in the *Tang Materia Medica* (*Tang Ben Cao*) (659 A.D.), and this herb probably arrived in China from India. In the Chinese tradition fennel is mainly used to move the Qi (especially through the liver) and to warm the kidneys and abdominal organs. Fennel is considered beneficial in all abdominal complaints (such as pains, indigestion, hernias and vomiting) that arise from coldness.

According to Ayurveda, fennel is a good herb for all constitutional types, balancing Vata, Pitta and Kapha, and promoting mental alertness. Because fennel is an excellent digestive tonic that can promote the digestive fire without aggravating Pitta, it is useful in all sorts of intestinal complaints, including colic and ulcer. In Ayurveda fennel is also employed in gynecology, since it promotes both a healthy menstrual flow and a nursing mother's flow of milk.

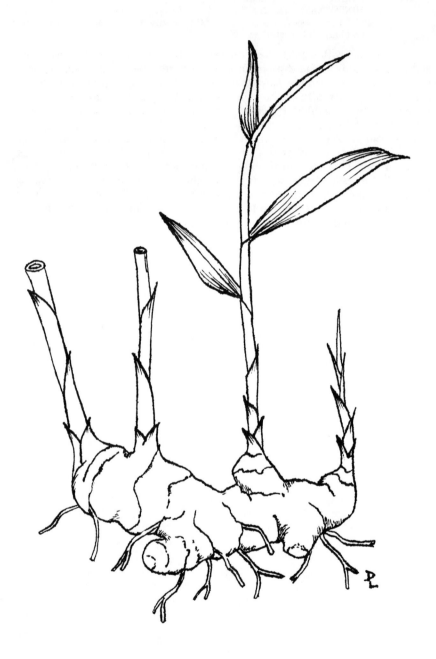

27. Ginger, *Zingiber officinale*

GINGER   BOTANICAL NAME: *Zingiber officinale*
              CHINESE NAME: gan jiang (dry), sheng jiang (fresh)
              SANSKRIT NAME: sunthi (dry), ardraka (fresh)
              PART USED: rhizome   TASTE: pungent & sweet   TEMPERATURE: hot

In the *Ramayana*, the revered Hindu scripture, a city is mentioned whose Sanskrit name was "ginger"; it was an important ginger trading center of the time. Ginger has been shipped since at least the second century B.C. from South India's Malabar Coast by both sea and land to Egypt, Arabia, Rome and the Mediterranean. Ginger is highly prized not only as a spice but also as a medicine; Ayurveda calls it "vishwabhesaja," the "universal medicine." It is considered one of the best and most Sattvic of herbs, and alleviates Vata and Kapha while only slightly aggravating Pitta. Generally, dry ginger is hotter and drier than the fresh; dry ginger reduces Kapha and promotes the digestive fire, while fresh ginger acts primarily on Vata but may be more aggravating to Pitta.

In Ayurveda ginger helps to regulate the whole alimentary tract, and is regarded such a strong digestive aid that it is given in such varied conditions as constipation, indigestion, vomiting, belching, flatulence, and dry hemorrhoids. Ginger has an equally beneficial effect upon the lungs, especially in respiratory infections, dyspnea, sore throat and cough, and edema. It is also applied externally, in certain types of rheumatic pains and headaches. One traditional Ayurvedic medicinal pill is made by mixing fresh ginger juice with ginger powder and rolling the combination into pea-size balls. This type of ginger pill, which thus combines virtues of both the dried and fresh forms, can control Kapha if it is mixed with honey, subdue Vata if combined with rock salt, and reduce Pitta if given with rock candy.

Ginger has been known and used in China since antiquity; Confucius is said to have eaten fresh ginger with each meal to improve his digestion. Many consider the plant to have come from the north, possibly Mongolia, on the basis of the etiology of the original character for ginger in the written language. Later on ginger became a commodity imported from India, as mentioned in the *Compendium of Materia Medica* under the name "celestial dried Indian ginger" (tian zhu gan jiang).

Chinese medicine teaches that both fresh and dried ginger have a powerful warming effect, with the dried form being slightly hotter than the fresh (which concurs with Ayurvedic opinion). Therapeutically, both forms of ginger are used to disperse coldness and promote sweating (as in the common cold or influenza), remove cold-phlegm lodged in the lungs (for coughs with thin sputum), alleviate coldness in the Middle Burner (which may cause stomach pains, chronic colitis, vomiting, indigestion, and so on), and dispel coldness trapped in the limbs (in cases of cold extremities and weak pulse). Fresh ginger is also used to reduce the toxicity of certain mushrooms and other herbs, such as aconite and pinellia, while dried ginger is used to stop chronic bleeding of various types (especially uterine hemorrhage).

Chinese medicine also uses ginger whose surface has been charred. This form of ginger has a bitter and astringent taste, and is slightly cooler in temperature than either the fresh or dried forms. This charred ginger mainly acts on the liver, and helps to relieve abdominal pain and discomfort due to coldness.

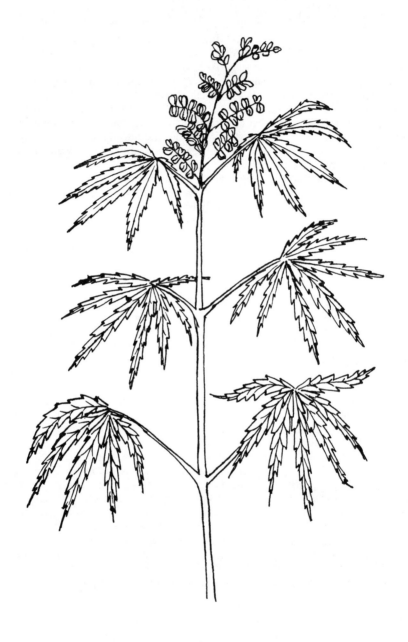

28. Hemp, *Cannabis sativa*

HEMP   BOTANICAL NAME: *Cannabis sativa*
       CHINESE NAME: huo ma   SANSKRIT NAME: vijaya
       PART USED: all parts   TASTE: bitter & sweet   TEMPERATURE: slightly warming

In China, there is a tradition which says that the second Emperor of the legendary era, the mystical Shen Nong who taught the people to cultivate the mulberry tree for raising silk worms, also taught them to cultivate hemp. Every part of the hemp plant was used medicinally in China: the male flowers to treat menstrual disorders, wounds and numerous other disorders that result from injury by the wind; the oil for hair loss, sulfur poisoning and throat dryness; the stalk as a diuretic and to expel urinary tract stones; and the juice of the root to expel a retained placenta or for post-partum hemorrhage. Although the leaves were considered poisonous, their freshly expressed juice was used to expel intestinal parasites and to neutralize the bite of a scorpion. The resinous female flowers were also considered poisonous; used in moderation they were held to calm the spirit, but, as Li Shi Zhen warns, when used in excess they "will produce hallucinations and unsteady the gait."

Currently the seeds are the most commonly used part of the plant in Chinese medicine, and the other parts are rarely employed. The seeds, which are considered to posses the sweet taste and to have a neutral temperature, are used mainly to moisten and nourish the intestines. They are thus useful in constipation, especially when the body's Yin becomes depleted (as it does with advancing age) or in cases of blood-deficiency (as seen in post-partum or surgical recovery). The seeds are used as an antidote to aconite and vermilion poisoning, and are said to help in maintaining the firmness of one's flesh. Externally the seeds are used to clear heat from sores and ulcerations.

That the ancient Chinese master of medicine Hua Tuo used a cannabis drink as a surgical anesthetic suggests, along with his remarkable surgical techniques which resemble those of the Indian surgeon Jivaka, that his knowledge came at least in part from Indian sources. India's most ancient book of healing lore, the *Atharva Veda*, mentions bhanga (Cannabis sativa) as one of five sacred (psychotropic) plants; another Sanskrit name for hemp is vijaya ("conquest"), because hemp grants victory to those who consume it. Of the three parts of the plant which are commonly used today in India (bhang, which is made from the leaves of both the female and male plants, and possibly from the male flowers also; ganja, which is the flowering tops of the female plants; and charas, the resin), only bhang and ganja are used in medicine. Bhang is often associated with seekers of religious ecstasy, and has been popularly used in temple celebrations and ceremonies since at least medieval times. One affectionate folk-name for Lord Shiva, the god of transformation, is in fact Bhangeri Baba ("Bhang-exhilarated Father").

In Ayurvedic medicine hemp is considered to be bitter and sweet, while having a slight heating quality. In small doses it can mildly aggravate Pitta while alleviating Kapha and Vata, but in large doses or when used over a long period of time it aggravates all Doshas. Hemp is rarely used alone in medicine, and its effects on the body vary according to the other herbs administered with it. With digestive herbs hemp can increase appetite, reduce nausea and abdominal distension, control diarrhea or relieve constipation; with aphrodisiac substances hemp itself becomes aphrodisiac; and when smoked with tobacco it suppresses the appetite and becomes anti-aphrodisiac. Given with Vata-controlling herbs hemp becomes an analgesic for headaches, abdominal spasms and neuralgia. More recently hemp has been found useful in alleviating the nausea and pain in cancer patients, and to reduce conditions of blood pressure and inter-ocular pressure (as in glaucoma). In such cases, Ayurveda recommends oral administration rather than inhaling smoke for greatest therapeutic efficacy.

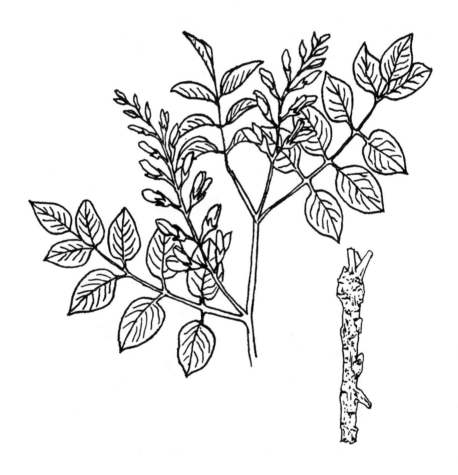

29. Licorice, *Glycyrrhiza glabra*

LICORICE   BOTANICAL NAME: *Glycyrrhiza glabra*
CHINESE NAME: gan cao   SANSKRIT NAME: yashtimadhu
PART USED: root   TASTE: sweet (c) / sweet & bitter (a)
TEMPERATURE: neutral (c) / cooling (a)

Licorice is one of the most important and frequently used plants in Chinese pharmacology because of its sweet taste and neutral temperature which gives it an ability to moderate and harmonize the characteristics of other herbs. Licorice is frequently utilized to modulate excessively hot or cold substances, and to mitigate or neutralize the violent properties of certain toxic substances. Furthermore, licorice is believed to help other substances penetrate to their appropriate destination in the tissues, with many an ancient and modern text claiming that it can enter all organs and Meridians. So common is the use of licorice that it appears in almost all prescriptions.

Chinese medicine teaches that licorice by itself strengthens both Qi and blood, and uses it to treat such symptoms as palpitations, shortness of breath, irregular pulse, and fatigue. Licorice is specific for most lung complaints (such as wheezing, sore throat, and cough), be they accompanied by either heat or cold symptoms. It is also specific for spasms in the abdomen or legs, in which case it is administered in the honey-fried form (which is considered then to be warm in temperature).

Ayurveda has long used licorice, and good-grade licorice was imported from Northern China and Mongolia during their long periods of contact. Ayurveda classifies licorice as cooling in temperature and as alleviating to both Pitta and Vata, though it can aggravate Kapha if used over a long time. Because licorice slightly increases body fluids, it is counter-indicated in Kapha disorders such as edema or hypertension (which agrees with Chinese medicine's prohibition of licorice in the presence of internal dampness). In large doses however licorice is used to induce vomiting, and to remove Kapha from the stomach and lungs thereby! It is this ability to increase body fluids which makes licorice a good aphrodisiac. Licorice extract made into lozenges is very popular in India even today to soothe the throat and to help relieve obstruction in breathing. It is also known to have a wonderful Sattvic quality which balances the mind and calms the spirit.

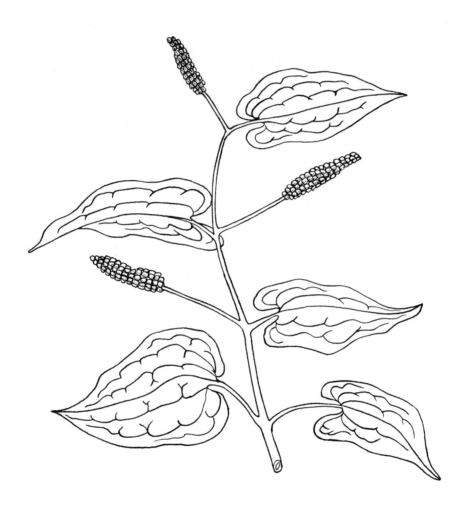

30. Long Pepper, *Piper longum*

LONG PEPPER   BOTANICAL NAME: *Piper longum*
CHINESE NAME: bi bo   SANSKRIT NAME: pippali
PART USED: fruit and root TASTE: pungent   TEMPERATURE: hot

In Ayurveda long pepper is considered a powerful digestive stimulant that increases digestive fire and reduces accumulation of digestive toxins (ama). Indeed, the *Charaka Samhita* praises the long pepper as being the best of all digestive stimulants. Historically, long pepper and its cousin black pepper were two of India's most important trade commodities, bringing many seafaring nations to the shores of the southern state of Kerala since Roman times or even before. Though pungent in taste, long pepper possesses a sweet post-digestive effect, which enables it to reduce both Vata and Kapha. Being strongly heating it removes internal cold and congestion. Long pepper is considered to be a rejuvenative and virilizer, an aphrodisiac which can regulate the sexual secretions due to its unctuous, sweet nature; its cousin black pepper, which is drying, has neither of these two effects.

Long pepper is traditionally used in digestive disorders like abdominal distension, ascites, diabetes, diarrhea, liver and spleen enlargement; in respiratory complaints like cough and asthma; and in rheumatic conditions. When used to enkindle the digestive fire, long peppers are often first soaked in salt water and then administered orally as a paste. When used as a nourishing agent, they are taken with ghee (clarified butter) and honey to treat consumptive disorders or anemia or to gain weight. The root is used almost exclusively to enkindle the digestive fire.

The Chinese name for this plant "bi po li" is given in the *Compendium of Materia Medica* as being an approximation of the Sanskrit "pippali" which came from the Buddhist lands of Magadhi (present day North India). Interestingly, the Chinese name for black pepper ("hu jiao") literally translates as barbarian pepper! This same text considered the root of this plant to be weaker in quality than the fruit, but not inferior in its action.

Clinically, in Chinese medicine, long pepper is mainly used to dispel coldness and warm the abdominal organs. It is therefore considered useful when coldness has lodged in the stomach and intestines (as in nausea, vomiting, belching and abdominal pain), uterine coldness (as in infertility), and bladder coldness (as in urinary tract infections).

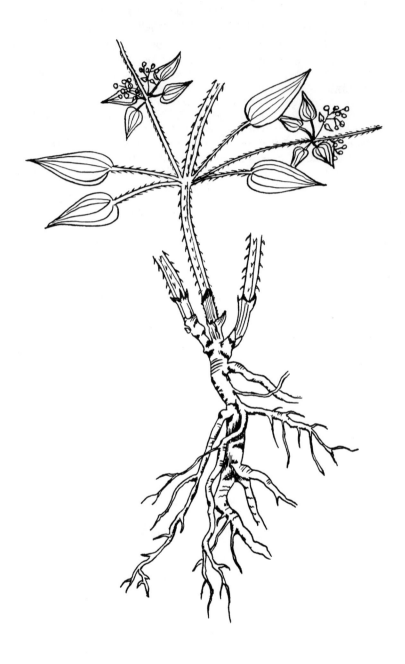

31. Madder, *Rubia cordifolia*.

MADDER   BOTANICAL NAME: *Rubia cordifolia*
CHINESE NAME: qian cao gen   SANSKRIT NAME: manjishta
PART USED: root   TASTE: bitter & sweet (a), bitter (c)
TEMPERATURE: cool

Madder is a prolific weed which grows throughout Asia. Perhaps early.man was first drawn to this plant by the deep red color of the root which was much used as a dye. In China since antiquity, madder was highly prized for its ability to rectify disorders of the blood. In the *Historical Records* (*Shu Jing*), an ancient text from the Spring and Autumn Period 770-476 B.C., it is stated that "he who plants a thousand mu (roughly two hundred acres) of this plant and gardenia is considered to be equal in rank to a nobleman who controls a thousand households."

In traditional Chinese medicine madder's cooling property is thought to counteract all kinds of bleeding conditions (from the nose, uterus, colon or respiratory tract) arising from heat-in-the-blood syndrome. Because madder also invigorates the blood and dispels blood flow stagnation, it is useful for various joint and muscular pains that arise from injuries, as also for contusions and fractures. Madder is also used for amenorrhea due to blood stasis. Modern Chinese research has shown madder to have antibacterial efficacy against both staphylococcus and streptococcus.

Ayurveda views madder as one of its most important Pitta-reducing and blood-purifying herbs, and uses it for conditions similar to those for which it is used in Chinese medicine. Ayurveda also uses madder to help mend broken bones, to treat toxic blood conditions such as genital herpes, jaundice, hepatitis and obstinate skin disorders, and to dissolve kidney stones and tumors in the body. It is also applied externally to inflamed or burned skin tissue.

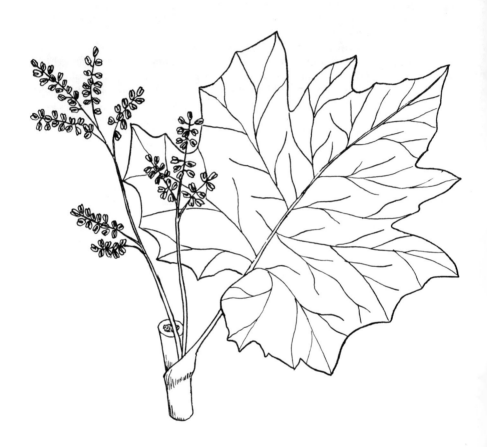

32. Rhubarb, *Rheum palmatum, Rheum emodi*

RHUBARB   BOTANICAL NAME: *Rheum palmatum, Rheum emodi*
CHINESE NAME: da huang   SANSKRIT NAME: amlavetasa
PART USED: root   Taste: bitter   TEMPERATURE: cold

Rhubarb has a long history in Chinese trade and medicine. Chinese rhubarb root produced in Shaanxi province was exported via the Silk Road as early as 114 B.C. This medicine became a much prized commodity throughout Eurasia, and particularly in Rome, Turkey, Russia and India. Rhubarb is mentioned in the late first century A.D. by Dioscorides, a Greek physician who served in the Roman army, in his *Materia Medica (Peri Hulas Iatrikos)*. Similarly rhubarb soon found a place in the Ayurvedic materia medicas. Marco Polo, the thirteenth-century Venetian traveler-merchant, imported the root into Europe. From roughly 1650 to 1780 Imperial Russia tried to monopolize the trade of rhubarb through a specially assigned "Rhubarb Office" at her frontier. This effort was partially successful, in the sense that rhubarb exported out of China from other ports was considered inferior in quality to that acquired and marketed by the Russians.

Since antiquity Chinese medicine has recognized and utilized rhubarb root's medicinal virtues; it considers the leaves to be poisonous. Raw rhubarb acts as a strong purgative on the gastrointestinal tract; when charred it can arrest bleeding; and when prepared with wine or vinegar it invigorates the blood. Rhubarb also removes heat and damp-heat symptoms in conditions such as jaundice, liver or gallbladder inflammation, dysentery, high fever, appendicitis, constipation, hemorrhoids, bleeding duodenal or intestinal ulcers, and painful urination. In consequence of rhubarb's blood invigorating effect it is used to treat immobile abdominal masses or localized pain due to blood stasis, amenorrhea, and hot, painful, sore eyes due to toxic liver fire.

Rhubarb is grown in many countries including India, although the original Chinese variety is still imported into India and sold in her bazaars under the name "revanda-chini." Ayurveda, like Chinese medicine, recognizes rhubarb as a purgative plant, using it almost exclusively for gastro-intestinal cleansing and regulation. Rhubarb reduces Vata (by channeling the wind downward through the intestines) and drains Pitta through its cooling nature. Rhubarb is considered to have a slightly astringent after-effect that protects the tone of the intestines, although it is rarely used alone because it can be too drying for the intestines. Externally a paste of the root is applied to reduce bruises and similar swellings.

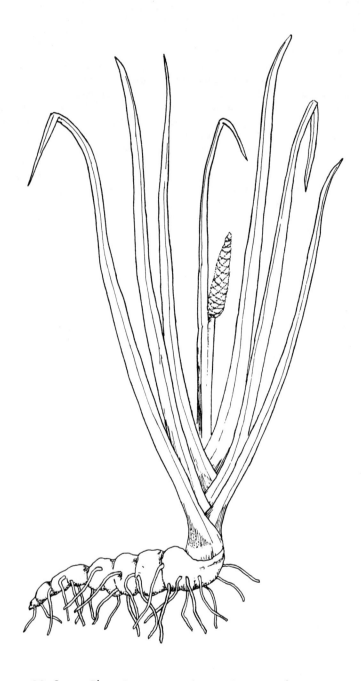

33. Sweet Flag, *Acorus gramineus, Acorus calamus*

SWEET FLAG   BOTANICAL NAME: *Acorus gramineus, Acorus calamus*
CHINESE NAME: shi chang pu   SANSKRIT NAME: vacha
PART USED: root   TASTE: pungent (c) / bitter & pungent (a)
TEMPERATURE: hot

In India the Acorus calamus variety of sweet flag has long been used since at least the Vedic period. In China various species of sweet flag have been used since ancient times (they find a place in the celebrated *Shen Nong's Materia Medica* of the later Han dynasty). Both traditions use sweet flag in similar ways.

In Ayurvedic medicine sweet flag is renowned for its rejuvenating and purifying effect upon the mind. Its Sattvic and warm nature helps to enhance memory and awareness, increasing mental vigor while simultaneously calming the mind. Sweet flag (also known as calamus), which calms Vata and Kapha while aggravating Pitta, is said to revitalize Prana and clear the subtle channels of toxins and obstruction, is especially beneficial in treating seizures. It is highly efficacious in treating sleepwalking, sleeptalking and bedwetting. It is suffused into the nostrils in powder form for nasal congestion and polyps, or to induce return of consciousness in cases of shock or coma. Externally, a paste is used to relieve headaches and insomnia. Sweet flag is also an antidote for the mental and physical side effects of cannabis and other mind-altering drugs, particularly when they are smoked or otherwise consumed together. Calamus also regulates breathing, relieves asthma, and helps expel phlegm from the lungs. Externally, it is used in massage oils to invigorate circulation and promote muscular relaxation.

In China a number of varieties of sweet flag are used, including Acorus gramineus, Acorus terrestris and Acorus calamus. Chinese medicine, perceives all these different species to contain the same therapeutic properties, and considers sweet flag as mostly aromatic. This signifies its ability to awaken the spirit and sensory orifices, especially when they are obstructed by the presence of phlegm (as in deafness, dizziness, forgetfulness, mental dullness, or seizures). Sweet flag is also used to dispel dampness that has become lodged in the chest or abdomen (as in asthma, chest pain and congestion, abdominal distension, or indigestion), and is also applied as a useful external remedy for musculoskeletal pains, trauma, and sores that are the result of cold, dampness or wind invasion.

CINNABAR   SCIENTIFIC NAME: cinnabaris (mercuric sulfide)
CHINESE NAME: zhu sha   SANSKRIT NAME: hingula
PART USED: whole   TASTE: sweet (c)/ all six tastes (a)
TEMPERATURE: cool (c)/ hot (a)

The use of cinnabar by Taoist alchemists in search of the elixir of immortality came into vogue in China during the Han dynasty. Their researches disclosed that cinnabar possesses the perfect balance of Yin and Yang (mercury and sulfur on a physical level) once it has been purified from its toxic crude form to a transformed state via an exacting process of nine-fold sublimation. Cinnabar played a key role in the Taoist's proto-chemistry experimentations, which also led to major discoveries of methods for neutralizing potent naturally-occurring toxins. This research benefited medicine by opening up a wide variety of previously toxic mineral, plant and animal substances for therapeutic use. Eventually much of this information was shared with Indian Tantric adepts who went on to master their own unique processes of chemical transformation. This Indianized art of proto-chemistry may have been the foundation of the Siddha system of medicine whose techniques have influenced Ayurveda. It is interesting to note in passing that today, the use and importance of minerals and metals in Ayurveda greatly exceeds their use in Chinese medicine.

Cinnabar in Chinese medicine is mainly used to calm and balance the mind and spirit for such conditions as insomnia, anxiety attacks, convulsions and restlessness. Due to its cooling nature, cinnabar also acts as a potent agent for clearing excess toxic heat from the body as evident in suppurative skin infections, mouth sores and snake bites.

In Ayurveda, most minerals are used in very refined forms which have been subjected to repeated incinerations that leave the end-product chemically inert and thus non-irritating to the tissues. Such mineral ash (bhasma) preparations have a powerful catalytic effect on the metabolic processes. Both the naturally-occurring cinnabar and artificially-prepared mercuric sulfide are considered ideal rejuvenator of the blood because it contains both mercury and sulfur, the primal minerals, which are used in treating a whole host of chronic diseases. Cinnabar, according to Ayurveda, also promotes the health of reproductive tissues and secretions and is used specifically, as in China, for obstinate skin disorders and certain types of poisonings. In terms of the Doshas, cinnabar alleviates both Pitta and Kapha; some say it can be mildly aggravating to Vata.

MUSK   BOTANICAL NAME: *Moschus moschiferus*
CHINESE NAME: she xiang   SANSKRIT NAME: kasturi
PART USED: preputial gland secretion of the musk deer
TASTE: pungent (c) / pungent and sweet (a)   TEMPERATURE: hot

Human beings for at least the last 2,500 years have been using the preputial glands of the musk deer for medicine and perfume. The best quality of musk reportedly becomes available during the rutting season when the animal breaks the gland's capsule with its hooves to empty the contents on to the ground, but this quality is extremely rare. Each capsule is said to contain up to 50 ml. of musk which has a milky texture and color when fresh but this gradually turns viscous and reddish-brown over time. Long ago the wild mountain musk deer roamed in large numbers throughout the Himalayas from Kashmir, Assam, Nepal, Tibet and into the Chinese provinces of Sichuan and Yunnan. Today it has become an endangered species, and wild musk has become difficult to obtain. Most commercially available musk is either synthetically produced or comes from musk deer farms.

The uses of musk are generally similar in both Ayurveda and Chinese medicine, though the specific conditions for which it is prescribed differ greatly. Because musk is highly regarded in Chinese medicine for its potent consciousness-reviving effect it is used to treat fainting, seizures, collapse, delirium, heart attacks, and traumatic injuries which cause mental shock and confusion. Musk's ability to awaken the mind and spirit is due to its intense aromatic and penetrating nature. Traditionally musk is also used to treat amenorrhea and hasten delivery including expulsion of retained placenta or facilitation of the downward passage of stillborn. Musk is used topically, in the form of a plaster (usually mixed with other herbs and beeswax), to treat traumas and injuries that result from nerve damage and painful conditions.

Musk is perhaps Ayurveda's most well known animal-derived product due to its powerful aphrodisiac effect, and which can markedly increase semen production in the male. Musk is said to alleviate Vata and Kapha while aggravating Pitta. Being both pungent and warming (as well as having a special vasodilator effect upon the blood vessels), musk stimulates the heart and blood circulation, and is thus considered a general tonic in cases of debility.

APPENDIX II
The Use of Vital Points in Asia

The practices of acupuncture and moxibustion, which use needles and mild cauterization respectively to stimulate the vital points along the energetic pathways called Meridians, are considered integral parts of traditional Chinese medicine. While a growing body of scientific evidence supports acupuncture's therapeutic claims, a scientific explanation for how acupuncture works still remains elusive. The origin of these treatments go back as far as the origin of Chinese Civilization itself, although historical evidence suggests that acupuncture and moxibustion arose separately and were slowly integrated over time. The ancients maintained that while acupuncture came from the eastern parts of China, moxibustion originated in the north, probably Mongolia. The merger of these two medical modalities into a single system occurred sometime during the Warring States period (475–221 B.C.). The basic philosophy of acupuncture and moxibustion is summarized in the *Yellow Emperor's Inner Classic*, which appeared during that era, and in the *Classic of Difficult Issues*, which was written during the Han Dynasty (206 B.C.–220 A.D.).

Both acupuncture and moxibustion have been refined and enlarged over the centuries, and in recent years acupuncture has "gone high tech" with the development of both laser acupuncture and electro-acupuncture. Most practitioners however continue to practice acupuncture and moxibustion, as well as the adjunctive techniques of acupressure, massage and micro-bloodletting in traditional ways, according to teachings based upon the laws of Yin-Yang and the Five Elements.

China is not alone in Asia in the use of vital points in therapy. Various indigenous systems have mapped such points on the body's surface, and assigned to them specific effects and uses. The most notable among these comparable traditions is the Indian concept of Marmas, which is discussed particularly in Ayurveda's most important surgical texts, the Sushruta Samhita. The Sri Lankan, Tibetan, and Mongolian healing traditions incorporate elements of either the Chinese or Indian concepts or both into their own distinctive ideas.

Marmas probably were first identified during the Vedic period, when kings and warriors may have used this science either to effectively inflict fatal wounds on their enemies (or animals of prey) or to prevent such wounds from becoming fatal. Sushruta, who teaches that every Marma is a seat of Prana, describes 107 Marmas on the surface of the human body. He states that when a Marma is traumatized, the destabilized Prana aggravates the body's Vata Dosha, which in turn blocks the Pervasive (vyana) Vata channels that circulate near the body's surface. Marmas are classified according to the underlying structure involved (muscles, blood vessels, ligaments, nerves, bones, joints), their regional location, their dimension, and the consequences of injury (swift death, death after some delay, death as soon as any foreign body is extracted from the wound, disability, or simply intense pain).

Knowledge of the Marmas was an integral part of Ayurvedic study, especially for surgery. Later physicians, such as Vagbhata and Sharngadhara (respectively of the 7th and 13th century A.D.), wrote commentaries on the Marma teachings of Sushruta. These ancient Indian doctors emphasized that the situation and dimension of each local Marma should be studied before any surgical operation, so that the incision could elude even the edge of a Marma thus avoiding further aggravation of the body's Prana. The use of certain external medicines (especially minerals or strong plants) were prohibited on Marmas.

In South India the practical application of Marmas was developed into a unique form of treatment called "marma-chikitsa" by Ayurvedic physicians, and "varma-kalai" by Siddha physicians. Practitioners of the martial art known as "kalarippayattu" in the state of Kerala use similar techniques. In the Southern tradition many of the same 107 Marmas are used, along with a number of special or secret Marmas, often unique to that practitioner's school of training. Therapeutically massage, finger pressure, medicated oils or mineral-vegetable poultices are applied to the individual Marmas. In the South Indian view, Marmas are considered to possess unique healing virtues because they intimately link with and thereby affect the body's Prana and Nadis. These properties of Marmas are therefore utilized to treat numerous ailments.

Bloodletting (siravedhividha) and cauterization (agnikarmavidhi) are frequently employed in India, although not to the 107 Marma points, for such conditions as hernias, hemorrhoids, and arthritic joints. Bloodletting is done directly to the superficial veins at precise locations along their pathways, and cauterization is applied by way of ignited plants, alkalis or special instruments either to specific points or directly to the disordered tissues. Bloodletting is generally used to dissipate excess heat and to cool the blood, while cauterization dispels coldness and heats the blood.

The Tibetan tradition of vital points basically modified and refined the Ayurvedic model to suit its concept of the body. The main distinctions between the two models are that the Tibetans used a greater number of points, and classified these into various types according to their use in bloodletting (gtar-dmigs), minor surgery (thur-dmigs), or cauterization (me-dmigs) points. Some, such as the vulnerable (gnad-dmigs) points, were prohibited for use. These differences are illustrated in the 17th century medical paintings of Sangye Gyamtso called the *Blue Beryl*, a series of 77 drawings depicting the essential medical teachings of the *Four Tantras*.

It is a curious fact that the Tibetans, who understood and borrowed many Chinese medical teachings (such as pulse diagnosis), did not adopt the techniques of Chinese acupuncture. Indeed, the *Blue Beryl* has no illustrations of any acupuncture points or instruments; it does show energetic pathways, but they differ from the Chinese Meridians in number and trajectory. Another anomaly: while the Chinese system of moxibustion uses mugwort almost exclusively as its cauterizing agent, the Tibetans apply (depending on symptoms) many other substances including gerbera, yellow champa, saffron, chebulic myrobalan, ginger and thistle.

Sri Lanka appears to possess an indigenous form of therapeutic acupuncture. Numerous documents on Sinhalese Buddhist and Ayurvedic medicine written on palm-leaf attest to the ancient use of fine acupuncture needles (22 recorded types), surgical lances for bloodletting, and cauterization on specific points (nilas) on the body's surface. The Sri Lankan vital points for acupuncture, bloodletting and cauterization surprisingly differ from the 107 Marmas of Ayurveda, but appear to be similar in their location to those of the Chinese system.

A study done by Laxman Devasena, entitled *Some Traditional Sri Lankan Medical Techniques Related to Acupuncture*, reveals a system of great breadth and long history. In Sri Lanka even today many practitioners use these ancient techniques both on humans and animals. According to Dr. V. Dharmalingam, there exists a small group of Siddha and Ayurvedic practitioners in South India who use gold and copper needles to acupuncture certain vital points. Apparently the long periods of mutually enriching contact between South India and Sri Lanka, which lie across the Palk Strait from each other, led to much medical cross-fertilization.

The concept of vital points in the Indian and Chinese traditions share many similar features overall:

  a) vital points are individually named and located through a system
     of precise anatomical measurement based on figure units,
  b) the points are situated on energetic pathways (Nadis or
     Meridians) in which Prana and Qi flow respectively,
  c) surgery, trauma or imbalance to a vital point (or Meridian, in
     the Chinese view) causes serious harm, and compromises health,
  d) a considerable number of Marma points correspond in location to
     the Chinese points (according to research done by Dr. D. G.
     Thatte; see his book *Acupuncture, Marma and Other
     Asian Therapeutic Techniques*),
  e) in both systems there is a comparable use of bloodletting and
     cauterization or moxibustion.

Important differences between Indian and Chinese views include the following:

  a) In the Ayurvedic tradition only 107 vital points are used, all
     of which are considered vulnerable points and thus unsuitable
     for therapy (except among those South India practitioners who

employ these and other points for healing). Chinese medicine describes more then 365 points for therapeutic use by puncture, cauterization, or bleeding.

b) Unlike the Marmas or Sri Lankan acupuncture points (nilas), the Chinese vital points are generally all linked together in a series of Meridians, which are in turn associated to specific organs and tissues.

c) Marmas are used, in the South Indian tradition mainly to treat disorders in their adjacent tissues or organs, whereas in China, acupuncture points are used for systemic effect and local use.

d) The various points mentioned in the Chinese, Indian, Sri Lankan and Tibetan systems rarely overlap.

GLOSSARY OF SANSKRIT AND CHINESE TERMS

CHINESE TERMS

These are the pinyin equivalents of Chinese characters. Tones are not indicated.

ba gang	eight guiding principles	tan	phlegm
hun	spiritual soul	wei	protective
jing	essence	wu	void
jing	meridians	wu xing	five elements
jinye	fluids	xin bao	heart protector
jiu	moxibustion	xue	acupuncture point
liu jing bing	six stages	xue	blood
liu yin	six pernicious influences	ying	nutritive
mai	vessels	yu xue	stagnant blood
po	animal soul	zang fu	organs
san jiao	triple burner	zang xiang	organ images
shen	spirit	zheng	acupuncture
tai yi	supreme ultimate	zong	ancestral

Qi. Denotes the inherent life force or bio-energy that animates the body. Qi, which exists in all living and non-living forms throughout creation, is differentiated according to its various functions and/or location.

Tao. Literally, "the way." In Chinese philosophy, the Tao denotes the unmanifest source of creation that gives rise to the Supreme Ultimate (tai yi) from which the universe unfolds.

Yang. The positive principle manifesting from nature's primal duality.

Yin. The negative principle manifesting from nature's primal duality.

SANSKRIT TERMS

ahamkara	ego	prabhava	powers
ama	digestive toxins	prakriti	nature
apana	downward-moving	purusha	reality
asthi	bone	rakta	blood
kosas	sheaths	rasa	sap
mahat	intelligence	samana	equalizing
majja	marrow	shukra	reproductive tissue
mamsa	flesh	srotamsi	channels
medas	fat	sushumna	central conduit
ojas	essence	tejas	subtle fire
pancha karma	five purifications	upana	upward moving
pancha mahabhuta	five elements	vyana	pervasive

Chakra. Literally, "a wheel." Chakras are sites where subtle aspects of consciousness gather along the body's main Nadi, the Central Conduit (sushumna).

Doshas. Literally, "fault or error, a thing which can go wrong." The Doshas in Ayurveda are grosser forms of Prana, Subtle Fire and Essence, which appear in the body as those condensations of the Five Great Elements known as Vata, Pitta and Kapha.

Kapha. The Dosha mainly associated with the Water principle.

Nadis. The subtle conduits through which Prana moves.

Marma. Literally, "a vital point or place." A Marma is a point on the human body beneath which the vital Nadis intersect.

Pitta. The Dosha mainly associated with the Fire principle.

Prana. The life force or energy which holds body, mind and spirit together, animating their functions. Prana, which also means breath, is closely associated with respiration, although oxygen is but one of its vehicles.

Rajas. One of the Three Great Attributes (gunas); it reflects a tendency towards activity, motion and lightness.

Sattva. One of the Three Great Attributes (gunas); it reflects a tendency towards equilibrium and subtleness.

Tamas. One of the Three Great Attributes (gunas); it reflects a tendency towards inertia and density of matter.

Vata. The Dosha mainly associated with the Air principle.

SOURCES OF ILLUSTRATIONS

6. Reprinted from *Systematic Classic (Lei Jing)*, by Zhang Jie Bin, 1624.

8. Drawing based on illustration in *Pratima-Kosha: Encyclopaedia of Indian Iconography*, Kalpatharu Research Academy, v.3, Bangalore, India, 1988.

9. Reprinted, by permission, from *Ayurveda: The Science of Self-Healing*, by Dr. Vasant Lad, p. 17.

10-11. Diagrams © 1995 N. Agarwal, Lotus Light Publications.

13. Reprinted courtesy of Robert Beer, from *Aghora II: Kundalini*, by Robert Svoboda, Albuquerque: Brotherhood of Life, 1993.

14. From the W.A. de Silva manuscript as shown in Laxman Devasena's, *Traditional Sri Lankan Medical Techniques Related to Acupuncture*, United Nations University, 1981, reprinted, by permission from the Marga Institute and United Nations University, Sri Lanka.

17. Reprinted, by permission, from *Bheshaja Kalpana-Pharmacology in Traditional Medicine*, Madras: Lok Swasthya Parampara Samvardhan Samithy, 1991.

18. Courtesy of Arnie Lade.

19. Reprinted, by permission, from *Marma Chikitsa in Traditional Medicine*, Madras, India: Lok Swasthya Parampara Samvardhan Samithy, 1991.

20. Reprinted, by permission, from *Tibetan Medical Paintings*, plate 22, London: Serindia Publications,1992.

22. Reprinted from *Systematic Classic (Lei Jing)*, Zhang Jie Bin, 1624.

23. Reprinted, by permission, from *Tibetan Medical Paintings*, plate 3, London: Serindia Publications, 1992.

24-33. © 1995 Diane Lade.

Book cover art: Hua Tuo reprinted courtesy of Arnie Lade, drawing of Dhanvantari based on illustration in *Pratima-Kosha: Encyclopaedia of Indian Iconography*, Kalpatharu Research Academy.

BIBLIOGRAPHY

Amber, R. and A. Babey-Brooke. 1966. *The Pulse: In Occident and Orient.* New York: Aurora Press.

Beinfield, H. and E. Korngold. 1991. *Between Heaven and Earth: A Guide to Chinese Medicine.* New York: Ballantine Books.

Bensky, D. and A. Gamble. 1993. *Chinese Herbal Medicine: Materia Medica.* Rev. ed. Seattle, WA: Eastland Press.

Chattopadhyaya, D. 1977. *Science and Society in Ancient India.* Calcutta: Research India Publications.

Cheng, X.N. ed. 1987. *Chinese Acupuncture and Moxibustion.* Beijing: Foreign Languages Press.

Chinese Academy of Sciences. 1983. compiled work of various authors. *Ancient China's Technology and Science.* Beijing: Foreign Language Press.

Clifford, T. 1984. *Tibetan Medicine and Psychiatry: The Diamond Healing.* York Beach, ME: Samuel Weiser, Inc.

Dash, B. 1978. *Fundamentals of Ayurvedic Medicine.* Delhi: Bansal & Co.

———. 1991. *Materia Medica of Ayurveda.* Delhi: B. Jain Publishers Ltd.

Devasena, L. 1981. *Some Traditional Sri Lankan Medical Techniques Related to Acupuncture: A Study of the Sugathadasa Samararatne Manuscript.* (courtesy of Marga Institute) Colombo: United Nations University.

Dharmalingam, V., M. Radhika, and A. Balasubramanian. 1991. *Marma Chikitsa in Traditional Medicine.* Madras: Lok Swasthya Parampara Samvardhan Samithy.

Donden, Y. 1986. *Health Through Balance: An Introduction to Tibetan Medicine.* Ithaca, NY: Snow Lion Publications.

Feng G.F. and J. English. 1972. *Lao Tsu-Tao Te Ching.* New York: Random House.

Filliozat, J. 1964. *The Classical Doctrine of Indian Medicine.* Delhi: Munshiram Manoharlal.

Foster, S. and C. Yue. 1992. *Herbal Emissaries: Bringing Chinese Herbs to the West.* Rochester, VT: Healing Arts Press.

Frawley, D. and V. Lad. 1992. *The Yoga of Herbs: An Ayurvedic Guide to Herbal Medicine.* Twin Lakes, WI: Lotus Press.

Fu, W.K. 1982. *Traditional Chinese Medicine and Pharmacology.* Beijing: Foreign Languages Press.

Heyn, B. 1987. *Ayurvedic Medicine.* Translated by D. Louch. Wellingsborough, United Kingdom: Thorsons.

Huard, P. and M. Wong. 1968. *Chinese Medicine.* New York: McGraw-Hill Book Company.

Jaggi, O.P. 1981. *History of Science, Technology and Medicine in India:*
Volume 2: Ayurveda: Indian System of Medicine
Volume 5: Yogic and Tantric Medicine
Volume 8: Medicine in Medieval India
Delhi: Atma Ram & Sons.
Jayasuria, A. 1978. *Principles and Practice of Scientific Acupuncture.*
Colombo: Lake House Book Publishers.
Junius, M. 1985. *The Practical Handbook of Plant Alchemy.*
Rochester, VT: Healing Arts Press.
Kaptchuk, T.J. 1983. *The Web That Has No Weaver: Understanding Chinese
Medicine.* New York: Congdon and Weed.
Lad, V. 1990. *Ayurveda: The Science of Self-healing.* 2nd ed.
Twin Lakes, WI: Lotus Press.
Lade, A. 1989. *Acupuncture Points: Images and Functions.*
Seattle, WA: Eastland Press.
Liu, Y.C. (chief editor). 1988. *The Essential Book of Traditional
Chinese Medicine:*
Volume 1: Theory
Volume 2: Clinical Practice
New York: Columbia University Press.
McGrew, R.E. 1985. *Encyclopedia of Medical History.*
New York: McGraw-Hill Book Company.
Nadkarni, A.K. 1982. *Indian Materia Medica.* Bombay:
Bombay Popular Prakashan.
Parifionovitch, Y., G. Dorje, and F. Meyer. 1992. *Tibetan Medical
Paintings: Illustrations to the Blue Beryl Treatise of Sangye
Gyamtso.* New York: Harry N. Abrams, Inc.
Patnaik, N. 1993. *The Garden of Life, An Introduction to the Healing
Plants of India.* New York: Doubleday.
Perry, L. 1980. *Medicinal Plants of East and South-East Asia.*
Cambridge, MA: MIT Press.
Raina, B.L. 1990. *Health Science in Ancient India.*
New Delhi: Commonwealth Publishers.
Reid, D. 1987. *Chinese Herbal Medicine.* Boston: Shambhala Publications.
Schatz, J., C. Larre and E. Rochat de la Vallee. 1986. *Survey of Traditional
Chinese Medicine.* Columbia, MD: Institute Ricci and Traditional
Acupuncture Foundation.
Smith, F.P. and G.A. Staurt. 1976. *Chinese Medicinal Plants.* Compiled by
Li Shih Chen. San Francisco: Georgetown Press.
Starobinski, J. 1964. *A History of Medicine.* New York:
Hawthorn Books, Inc.
Svoboda, R.E. 1992. *Ayurveda: Life, Health and Longevity.*
New York: Penguin Books.
————. 1988. *Prakruti: Your Ayurvedic Constitution.* Albuquerque, NM:
Geocom.

Takakusu, J. 1956. Observations of Medicine in India and China - I
    Tsing. In *History of Science in India*. Edited by
    D. Chattopadhyaya. New Delhi: Editorial Enterprises.
Thatte, D.G. 1988. *Acupuncture, Marmas and Other Asian Therapeutic
    Techniques*. Delhi: Chaukambha Oriental Publishers.
Tierra, M. 1992. *Planetary Herbology*. Twin Lakes, WI: Lotus Press.
Tsarong, T.J. 1981. *Fundamentals of Tibetan Medicine According to
    the Rgyud-Bzhi*. Dharamsala, India: Tibetan Medical Center.
Udupa, K.N. and R.N. Singh, ed. 1978. *Science and Philosophy of Indian
    Medicine*. Nagpur, India: Shree Baidyanath Ayurved Bhawan Ltd.
Unschuld, P.U. *Medicine in China Series:*
    Volume 1: A History of Ideas. 1985
    Volume 2: A History of Pharmaceutics. 1986
    Berkeley: University of California Press.
Vieth, I. 1949. *The Yellow Emperor's Classic of Internal Medicine*.
    Berkeley: University of California Press.
Xie, Z.F. and X.K. Huang, ed. 1984. *Dictionary of Traditional
    Chinese Medicine*. Hong Kong: The Commercial Press, Ltd.
Zimmer, H.R. 1948. *Hindu Medicine*. Baltimore: Johns Hopkins Press.
Zimmermann, F. 1987. *The Jungle and the Aroma of Meats: An Ecological
    Theme in Hindu Medicine*. Berkeley: University of California Press.

INDEX

G

Ginger 127
Ginseng 40, 119
Golden Age of Buddhism 85
Guan Yin, Goddess of Mercy 87
Gunpowder 91

H

Heart Protector 23, 24
Hemp 83, 129
Hippocratic school 87
Hua Tuo 38, 83, 129
Hydrology 94

I

Inner Classic
    10, 25, 29, 37, 41, 80, 142
Integration of systems
    acupuncture 114
    adjunctive practices 114
    general outline 113
    Internal Medicine 114
    Purification therapy 115
Intelligence 47
Internal Medicine, Ayurveda
    administration 77
    formulas 77
    minerals 77
    theory 76
Internal Medicine, Ayurveda
    Vehicle 76
Internal Medicine, Chinese
    art of formulation 40
    direction of action 39
    five tastes 39
    formulas 40
    temperature 38
Internal Medicine,
    comparative view 108

J

Jivaka 85, 89

K

Kalarippayattu 61, 85, 143
Kapha 50, 76

L

Lao Zi 12
Law of Like and Unlike 50
Law of Microcosm and Macrocosm 49
Li Shi Zhen 119
Licorice 131
Long Pepper 133

M

Madder 135
Marmas 61, 88, 94, 142
    South Indian tradition 143
Massage 42, 76, 83, 114, 142
Mercury 91
Meridian System
    acupuncture and moxibustion 29
    ancient influences 94
    eight Extraordinary Vessels 27
    functions 25
    history 29
    point openings 28
    Qi flow through 25
    twelve Regular Meridians 25
    types of pathways 25
Moxibustion 29, 41, 88, 114, 142
    in Tibetan tradition 144
Musk 141

N

Nadis 60, 61, 83, 92, 143
Nalanda University 46, 88
Nature 47, 82
Nilas 88, 144

O

Organ functions
    Chinese view 23
    comparative view 97
Organ Images 21

P

Pernicious Influences 30, 87
Phlegm 31, 104
Pitta 50, 76
Post-digestive effect 51
Prana
    absorption of 99

AYURVEDIC COOKING FOR WESTERNERS

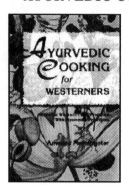

**Familiar Western Food
Prepared with Ayurvedic Principles**
by Amadea Morningstar
This book opens Ayurveda to everyone whether using Indian or Western ingredients, with more than 230 new and delicious recipes. Amadea Morningstar is co-author of *The Ayurvedic Cookbook,* the all time best-selling manual for applying Ayurveda to nutrition.

"*Ayurvedic Cooking For Westerners* holds together so harmoniously because of the author's generous gift of herself . . .As a reader, you will feel comfortable and at home in Amadea's earthy and healthy kitchen. Step right in." **Rebecca Wood,** author of *Quinoa the Super Grain*

416 pages pb $19.95
ISBN 0-914955-14-4

AYURVEDA SECRETS OF HEALING

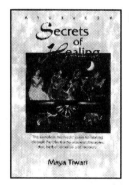

The complete Ayurvedic guide to healing through Pancha Karma seasonal therapies, diet, herbal remedies and memory.
by Maya Tiwari
The author is the first to reveal sophisticated and timeless processes of the original and rejuvenative therapies, including Panchakarma, first taught and practiced by the ancient Vedic seers, and readily adaptable to modern life.
"*Secrets Of Healing* is an authoritative compendium on the ancient wisdom and knowledge of healing that will be of immense value to health professionals as well as those who are interested in healing themselves."
Deepak Chopra, M.D., author of *Ageless Body,*
Timeless Mind

500 pages pb $22.95
ISBN 0-914955-15-2

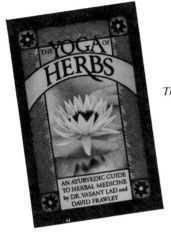

THE YOGA OF HERBS

by Dr. David Frawley and Dr. Vasant Lad

The Yoga of Herbs is a complete and detailed guide to herbal therapies, against the background of Ayurvedic medical theory and practice. This handbook is a must for the beginning and/or practising herbalist.

225 pages pb $12.95
ISBN 0-941524-24-8

LOST SECRETS OF AYURVEDIC ACUPUNCTURE

by Dr. Frank Ros

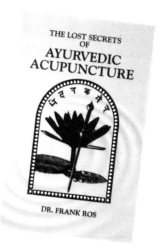

Dr. Ros has researched the ancient texts of Ayurveda to uncover the practice of acupuncture, pre-dating even the Chinese. He shows how acupuncture developed, including interesting insights useful to the modern-day practitioner, and discusses correspondences to Chinese medical practice.

232 pages   pb $15.95
ISBN 0-914955-12-8

PRAKRUTI

Your Ayurvedic Constitution

by Robert Svoboda

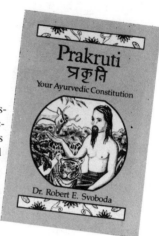

Ayurveda is the ancient healing science of India. It distinguished various body-types having distinct characteristics. Predilection to specific types of disease, as well as response to various types of treatment, is based on the constitutional type. This book is an excellent introduction to the science of Ayurveda.

206 pages pb $12.00
ISBN 0-945669-00-3

PLANETARY HERBOLOGY

by Michael Tierra
(edited by David Frawley)

From the best-selling author of *The Way of Herbs*
—more than 175,000 copies sold.

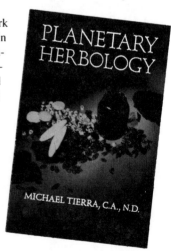

This practical handbook and reference guide is a landmark publication in this field. For unprecedented usefulness in practical applications, the author provides a comprehensive listing of the more than 400 medicinal herbs available in the west, classified according to their chemical constituents, properties and actions, indicated uses and suggested dosages. Students of Eastern medical theory will find the Western herbs cross-referenced to the Chinese and Ayurvedic (Indic) systems of herbal therapies. This is a useful handbook for practitioners and readers alike.

400+ pages, 51/2 x 81/2 $17.95
charts and illustrations
ISBN 0-941524-27-2

ADDRESSES
and SOURCES of SUPPLY

Fragrances, Gemstones, Herbs, Books and Cassettes

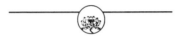

WHOLESALE
Contact with your business name,
resale number or practioner license.

LOTUS LIGHT ENTERPRISES, INC.
Box 1008 TD
Silver Lake, WI 53170
Voice 414/889-8501 • Fax 414/889-8591

RETAIL
LOTUS FULFILLMENT SERVICE
33719 116th Street Box TD
Twin Lakes, WI 53181

ABOUT THE AUTHORS

Arnie Lade is an acupuncturist practising in Victoria, British Columbia where he lives with his wife and children. He studied Chinese language at the University of Victoria and Xiamen University, and acupuncture and oriental medicine at the Beijing and Chengdu Colleges of Traditional Chinese Medicine in China. He is also the author of *The Acupuncture Points: Images & Functions*, a standard teaching text in its field, and is
a contributing author of *Chinese Massage Therapy*. Mr. Lade lectures widely
and is currently on the faculty of the Centro de Estudos de Medicina Oriental de Brasilia in Brazil.

Robert Svoboda graduated from the Tilak Ayurvedic College of the
University of Poona in 1980 as the first and, and until today, the only
Westerner ever to become a licensed Ayurvedic physician. Since then he
has travelled extensively, lecturing and conducting workshops on
Ayurveda. Among his writings are *Prakruti: Your Ayurvedic Constitution* and
Ayurveda: Life Health and Longevity. Mr. Svoboda is on the staff of the
Ayurvedic Institute in Albuquerque, New Mexico, and divides his time
principally between North America, Hawaii and India.

ACUPUNCTURE POINTS: IMAGES & FUNCTIONS
by Arnie Lade

An in-depth discussion of the derivation and clinical applications of hundreds of the
most commonly used acupuncture points. In this richly-researched book prepared in
consultation with leading Chinese scholars, Mr. Lade provides the images and functions, location, classifications, indications and contraindications for each of the points.
An extensive repertory of traditional functions and patterns with their associated
points enables the practitioner to move quickly from diagnosis to prescription of
appropriate points.
There is also a Chinese character dictionary which defines the Chinese characters
used in identifying point names. In addition, an index is included in which points are
arranged by channel, alphanumeric number, pinyin, and English for easy reference.
364 pages, 6x9 hb cloth $29.50
original brush calligraphy
ISBN 0-939616-08-4

To order: contact EASTLAND PRESS
1260 Activity Drive, Suite A
Vista, CA 92083
ph. 800/453-3278